This book champions a positive outlook on older age and seeks to show how later adulthood is more than a time of ill-health, decline, and disability, but rather a time rich with new experiences, adventures, and renaissance in our being. It takes an in-depth look into the creative expressions of people at midlife and in older age to discover ways to stay engaged, effectively cope, and realize personal growth and self-actualization. Stories and interviews from everyday people as well as professional and nonprofessional artists, musicians, poets, and writers are presented. There is also discussion of age-related and pathological changes in health, the utility of integrative art therapies, processes of resilience and growth, and the personal renewal that one may experience at midlife and in older age. Writing in an engaging style, the authors hope the reader will discover and continue to travel upon various creative pathways where they can find new opportunities for self-discovery, joy, and fulfillment in later life.

* * *

"'Celebrating the Arts of Living' invites the reader to consider the intrinsic value of the arts and their expression as part of life. Whether reading or writing poetry, listening to or performing music, or finding fulfillment in an activity like sailing, 'Celebrating' explores the human benefits of our involvement. In a society that often determines an activity's worth based on its commercial value, this book reveals merits in terms of holistic personal achievement and fulfillment."

   – Keith Davis, Bachelor of Music Education, Master of Science in Computer Science

"'Celebrating the Arts of Living' underscores the creative potential of aging and older age. It serves as a prolegomenon to a more fully realized paradigmatic shift in the social sciences and humanities to describe aging as it is experienced - rather than as it is assumed to be. The authors reframe our understanding of age-related changes in physical and cognitive health. In doing so they suggest health threats and the proximity to the end of life, rather than leading to prolonged despair, become springboards for deep, sustained appreciation and creativity. Throughout the book, engrossing life stories and accessible descriptions of research about the arts and creativity convey the increased richness of crystallized intelligence and empowering relationality of older age. From music making to arts-based movement, to writing and gardening, 'Celebrating the Arts of Living' recognizes and, indeed, celebrates the depth and breadth of being, especially in later life."

   – K. Jill Fleuriet, Ph.D., Professor of Anthropology, University of Texas at San Antonio

"Life is Art! Wonderfully expressed through a holistic and humanistic lens, 'Celebrating the Arts of Living' is a wonderful addition to the expanding world of arts in health resources. This book connects with the reader through its relatable, honest, and colorful life stories, that confront the process of aging with and through the arts - opening doors to deeper relationships, stronger resilience, new opportunities, challenges, and an embrace of life and its changes. It asks the questions, what is our story and what have we brought into existence? Finally, I commend the accessibility of this book, communicating directly and clearly to the broadest audience possible through chapters divided into short sections each expressing a complete idea or concept to inspire and renew hope."

- J. Todd Frazier, Composer and the Gerald H. Dubin, M. D. Presidential Distinguished Centennial Director in the Art of Medicine at Houston Methodist Hospital's System Center for Performing Arts (CPAM)

"This is a much-needed book as Professors VonDras and Madey address an often-overlooked perspective in aging—one that supports a balanced, creative, enjoyable, and fulfilling life. Through stories of real people, the book is reader-friendly and can help readers to uncover life meanings that are in constant development through the entire lifespan. The spirit of humanity is unveiled through connections, continuation, and creative expressions of all forms."

- C. Victor Fung, Ph.D., Professor of Music Education, University of South Florida

"Many seniors have come to regard aging as synonymous with loss. This book, carefully researched and full of personal experiences challenges that assumption, and instead shines a beacon of hope that there is much to celebrate and be enthused about in one's senior years. 'Celebrating the Arts of Living: Pathways to Joy and Fulfillment in Later Life' encourages the reader to become reacquainted with the joys that the arts can bring, be it music, writing, painting or something special that brightened our younger days, thus helping us to thrive and see such reawakening as a pathway to ongoing joy and fulfillment in our senior years."

 – Beverly Hays, Retired Nurse

"Expanding on their earlier scholarship on music, wellness and aging, Professors VonDras and Madey offer a thoughtful examination of creative arts involvement as a conduit to a more positive aging. A joy to read, the book offers a 'mental vitamin' for readers via an exploration of empirical research findings on the value of creative arts in treating aging-related wellness issues, and through the real-life stories of resilient older adults whose arts involvement sustained them in times of challenge, enhanced their well-being, and enriched their lives. A must-read for those interested in celebrating life in older adulthood!"

 – Lisa J. Lehmberg, Ph.D., Professor of Music Education,
   University of Massachusetts Amherst, USA

"A powerful testimony to the potential for personal growth and creativity in later life. The authors combine a wide-ranging survey of humanistic perspectives on the process of ageing, with powerful life stories drawn from the experiences of older people themselves. The book represents a unique account of the possibilities for self-discovery and self-expression in older age, providing an inspirational and visionary account of benefit for the scholar and layperson alike."

 – Chris Phillipson, Ph.D., Emeritus Professor of Sociology and
   Social Gerontology, University of Manchester, UK

"Like a beautiful piece of tapestry, this book weaves together a myriad of inspiring narratives about facing life challenges and the resilience of the human spirit. It places these stories in the context of modern research and theories as well as the wisdom traditions from cultures around the world. The authors' realistic but dignified outlook on later life makes readers look forward to how they will mature and to their future adventures. This was a pure delight to read!"

– Toru Sato, Ph.D., Professor of Psychology, Shippensburg University

"This beautifully written and richly rewarding book is like an eye-catching tapestry of contrasting colours capturing the paradox and duality of aging – both physical decline and spiritual growth, satisfaction, joy, and painful losses, death of the old self and regeneration of the best self. Through memorable stories of both world-renowned individuals and ordinary people, 'Celebrating the Arts of Living' opens our eyes to new vistas of life in later years and reveals the magic of the arts in everyday life that can transform and regenerate our lives. I highly recommend this book to not only students and professionals, but all individuals interested in wellbeing and authentic living across the lifespan."

– Paul T. P. Wong, Ph.D., C. Psych., Professor Emeritus, Trent University, President of the International Network of Personal Meaning

* * *

CELEBRATING THE ARTS OF LIVING: PATHWAYS TO JOY AND FULFILLMENT IN LATER LIFE

BY

DEAN D. VONDRAS, PH.D.

AND

SCOTT F. MADEY, PH.D.

TABLE OF CONTENTS

Preface to the Celebration of the Arts of Living

In later life, what spurs our creativity and what is acted out, re-told, sung, painted, sewn, sculpted, and understood, reflects a more mature orientation, and reveals deeper aspects of our living. Indeed, our creative expressions suggest new opportunities for personal discovery and revitalization. Further, later adulthood is more than a time of ill-health, decline, and disability, but rather a time rich with new experiences, adventures, and renaissance in our being. One example of this robust and triumphant older age is noted in the life of the writer George Sand, as Rene Doumic describes: "Nearly every year she went to some fresh place in France to find a setting for her stories… "I shall be turning my wheel when I die," she used to say… She celebrated the hymn of Nature, of love, and of goodness in it."[1] Like George Sand, in later life we too may continue to be creative, to celebrate Nature's hymn, songs of love, and all the goodness we may find in our living.

In this book, we seek to recognise the arts as pathways to joy and fulfilment in later life. Thus, we take an in-depth look into the creative expressions of people at midlife and in older age to discover ways to stay engaged, effectively cope, and realize personal growth and self-actualization. We present stories and interviews from everyday people as well as professional and nonprofessional artists, musicians, poets, and writers. We also include research describing age-related and pathological changes in health, the utility of integrative art therapies, processes of resilience and growth, and the personal renewal that one may experience at midlife and in older age.

Reasons for Writing This Book

Following upon our earlier work, *Music, Wellness, and Aging: Defining, Directing, and Celebrating Life*, we hope to further expand on the role of creativity in the celebration of life.[2] We believe that it is through our personal stories and the arts (singing, playing an instrument, painting, sculpting, etc.) that we connect to a profound sense of being that offers us hope and sustains us in our living. That in our creative activities we uncover the most essential aspects of what it means to be human. Moreover, in our creative expressions we often depict the key existential concerns that we confront in life. Thus, whether it is through art-making, dancing, playing a musical instrument, sewing, storytelling, or other creative activity, we may discover a new way of being and of seeing ourselves in later life.[3]

A second reason to write this book is to provide insight into the interdependencies we recognize when we consider one's involvement in a creative activity, its potential to move us in new ways and shape our living experience, and its influence on health and well-being. In doing so, we hope to show how later life is more than a time of ill-health, decline, and disability, but rather as a time of personal renaissance. A time where through our creative involvements we may rekindle earlier interests, reimagine what is possible, and discover new areas of personal growth.

A third reason we wrote this book is with the layperson in mind. A large body of literature on the topics of aging and creativity has been directed toward a specialized scientific audience. Thus, in contrast, we hope to include both the lay reader and the specialist in considering how one's participation in various creative activities may lead to joy and fulfillment in later life. Further, through our presentation of research, personal narratives, and stories of others, we hope to spur the reader's interest and involvement in creative activities that enhance their well-being and celebration of living.

* * *

About the Authors

This book is an outgrowth of both authors' creative interests and scholarly focus. Dean D. VonDras holds a B.A. in music and a Ph.D. in psychology. He plays piano, trumpet, and sketches. He is currently professor of psychology at the University of Wisconsin–Green Bay, where his research and teaching focus on adult development, health, and aging.

Scott F. Madey is an emeritus professor of Psychology at Shippensburg University and holds a Ph.D. in psychology. His research and teaching have focused on the history of psychology, multicultural health psychology, psychology of music, and the social psychology of aging. He also plays a variety of musical instruments such as guitar, French horn, and Eb alto horn. For over 20 years, he has been involved in the local town band, and ancillary offshoots such as the swing band and German band. He also plays jazz in a duo consisting of guitar and trombone and composes his own music.

ACKNOWLEDGEMENTS

We wish to thank reviewers of earlier chapters for their helpful comments and suggestions.

A very special thanks is also extended to the following:

Rebecca Mack who created a scrapbook about Helen Keller, and The American Foundation for the Blind for permission to reproduce and use works by Helen Keller, and the news article from "Scrapbook of Helen Keller and The Blind. Book XXXVII." Created by Rebecca Mack c... May 3, 1950 (afb.org);" Copyright © American Foundation for the Blind, Helen Keller Archive.

Molly B., Joseph B-L., Faith G., Ashley H., Dylan J., Hannah J., Gracie L., Trisha L., Isabella M., Kendall, R., Riley S., Austin S., Jasmine S., Paige S., and Amber T. for permission to use excerpts from their brief narrative essay on caricature drawing, May-December, 2021.

Rick Belcher and Meryl Shechter for permission to include excerpts from their life story interviews, September, 2020—May, 2021.

Bill Bowman, Managing Editor, of *The Daily Item* in Sunsbury, PA, for permission to reproduce and use the article, "Confidently Climb the Stair," May 3, 1950.

Victoria Jicha for permission to use excerpts from her life story essay and interview, October-November 2020, and from her article, "If I Only Knew Then What I Know Now" that appeared in *Flute Talk*, November, 2020.

Eileen Johnson for permission to use excerpts from her life story essay, May 24, 2021.

Participants in the Life Story Project conducted by Dean D. VonDras.

Joanne S. Rupp for permission to include and reproduce her poem, "Relevant Last Wishes," May 19, 2021.

Dr. Robert G. Santee for permission to use excerpts from his interview survey on Tai-Chi and Qigong practices, May 26, 2021.

The Smithsonian American Art Museum for permission to use *Virgen de los Caminos*, 1994, by Consuelo Jiminez Underwood.

Consuelo Jiminez Underwood for permission to use excerpts from her life story interview, April 4, 2021.

Benjamin Uribe-Cruz for permission to use excerpts from his family history essay, May 21, 2021.

Mitch Wadley for permission to include excerpts from his life story interview, August 16, 2020, and May 24, 2021, and to use lyrics from "Little Red Riding Hood (Featuring the Paper Bag)."

Jim Weatherhead for permission to use excerpts from his life story essay and poem, July 5, 2020.

Brother A. Brian Zampier for permission to use excerpts from his life story interview and *Sketch-Journal*, September 8, 2021.

We also thank our teachers, colleagues, and most importantly our students whose influence continues to direct and inspire us and have made this work possible. We similarly express great gratitude to our parents, brothers and sisters, nieces and nephews, and our entire family, whose love and support is deeply appreciated and resonates in our writing of this book.

Lastly, very special thanks go to Paula Madey, and Mary Elizabeth and Jack VonDras, for their sustaining love and encouragement throughout this project, and in our journey in life together.

Dean D. VonDras and Scott F. Madey

ONE — TOWARDS A CELEBRATION OF THE ARTS OF LIVING

A beloved Uncle recently sent me a brief family history. After the passing of his elder sister, he noted that he was the last of his siblings, and he did not want these stories to become lost to our family. Lovingly expressed, a family history recognizes the coming together of people, their cultural backgrounds, sites of origin and immigration, and the generational contributions of parents, grandparents, aunts and uncles, and others. It provides us a way to know extended family members, and gain insight into our collective hopes and concerns, the hardships and crises confronted, and how different events may have influenced our direction in life.

Often too, a family history can omit important pieces of information. It can leave out reasons for immigration, how couples met and formed families, reactions to social inequalities, or how challenges brought on by two world wars, world-wide terrorism, pandemics, and economic collapses were endured and overcome. Part of this loss is that often older family members never talked about their experiences, or information and documents may have become lost, or the family historian may have died before passing on to others the stories about the family's past.

As we reflect on our family histories, we may think of a fun uncle, a grandfather we never met, and feel love and joy, or tearful feelings of missing them or never knowing them. One author recalls his uncles who fought in WWII: One bayonetted in April 1945, very near the end of the war in Germany, but survived; another uncle who was at Pearl Harbor on December 7, 1941; another who was in the United States Army Signal Corps in Germany; and an uncle who fathered an American-German child there. There is a wish now to be able to talk to them, to parents, and others, but one can only imagine or infer from reading the history of those times or studying old maps and letters to fill in the blanks of history. As we recall the experiences of these uncles there are questions about what their thoughts were as they entered battle, how one felt about the child and mother he had left behind, and how they handled "memories" of war. They never talked about the war, and when asked would say, "you do not want to hear what happened." We may also recall the good times, the weddings, and reunions as well. There is the recollection of an aunt and uncle who were engaged for 14 years before finally getting married. Thoughts about a grandfather—a coal miner—who played the bass fiddle. Remembrances of one's mom who sang with a big band when younger. Reflectively, it seems that stories about moms, seem to be the story of "every mom." The story of miners and soldiers in our families is the account of every miner—every soldier. We all share commonalities. We raise families, watch loved ones grow and die, experience hardships and good times. Although the specifics of each person's story vary, we all share something central—our humanity. How we live our lives is our personal testament and expression of our connection to others. We realize in our family stories the purposeful and loving act of creating a shared and collective remembrance—and the importance of retaining a family's historical record. We understand too, like the poem "To Old Age" by Walt Whitman, that as we continue in our development into later life, we have new powers to reflect upon where we have been, and to look toward the future.[1] We see in our family histories the expanding and flowing river of life that we travel on, and their reflections that spread into an ever-wider sea of personal discovery and celebration of our living.

Life Story, Aging, and Creativity

This book considers three interconnected aspects of our human experience: Our life story, our aging, and our creativity. It is a book that champions a humanistic study of older age, and that seeks to show how these interrelated aspects may influence how we become in the second half of the life course. Moreover, it is a book that reveals a journey into a deeper and more profound psychology in older age – one of new identity and continuing search for meaning and purpose in our living.

Our life stories reflect our basic human need for self-expression. Through our personal narratives we announce our identity and connections to community. Our life stories intersect with another important concern explored in this book, and that is our perceptions and reactions to getting older. From our earliest moments in life, we have been involved in processes of transition and becoming. Moreover, since childhood we have been telling our story of growing and changing, of events and happenings encountered in adolescence and young adulthood, and of experiences we have come upon or will perhaps meet in middle or later life. Thus, more certain than taxes, and as inevitable as that other certainty, death, we continue to tell the story of our lives, and the changes that we encounter as we grow older. However, an important question we seek to address is how do we approach this inevitability? What story will we create about our personal experience of growing older? Do we view older age with dread and foreboding, or with anticipation and excitement, and as a time where we can creatively write new chapters in our book of life? Thus, a related third aspect we explore is our creativity—that basic drive to bring something into existence.

Coupled with our need to create, we also recognize the co-occurrence of our need for self-expression and other deeper psychological influences. Consequently, it is noted that our life stories are creations of our own. Further, we recognize that our interpretations of aging and creative impulses are interrelated and inseparable. Indeed, these three aspects of our human experience represent a conceptual whole. Thus, through our creativity, whether in our storytelling, music, needlework, painting, dancing, other arts, crafts and hobbies, or through immersive experiences when we visit an art museum or attend a concert, we respectively construct and encounter an intricate mosaic that tells of our life. In this introductory chapter and those that follow, we will further discuss this interconnectedness of life story, aging, and creativity as it may lead us to discover enjoyment and celebration in our living.

Importance of Each Person's Life Story

As put forth by Jan Baars, there is an art of living made accessible through the life stories of older adults.[2] Indeed, it is only through listening to the person and how they understand the world that we gain insight into their life. We add that it is only through seeking and recognizing the creative expressions, personal accounts, and insights of older people that we may come to understand the uncertainties and crises that arise in later life, and find new insights and diverse interpretations of what it means to grow older. Like the older adult with dementia who still attends an occasional hockey game with family members, when we seek to listen to and understand the older person's current experiences, we can discover many new insights and interpretations of what it means to mature and grow older. In the personal narratives of older people, we realize a more human expression of the ongoing processes and experiences of later life. Further, by listening to a person's story in a caring way, we have the opportunity to hear and ponder wisdoms that may illuminate and aid our own living. Thus, as Carl Jung has alluded, perhaps we too will recognize that it is in the last half of the life course, those years from our 40s and beyond, where one may become involved in life's greatest adventures, experience new opportunities for self-discovery and creative expression, and make one's greatest contributions to family and to community.[3]

In many ways, each person's life can be described as a great book. It includes many chapters, with vivid scenes and intriguing plots, and often with an accompanying reflective dialogue of personal meaning that makes the saga of one's life story richer and more complex as one chapter closes and a new chapter begins. Certainly, as we listen to older family members and friends, we recognize the gift of drinking in the narrative and finding a profound meaning in their stories. As we come to understand their interest in songs from a specific time of history, or reason for composing a poem or painting, or in their self-expression that is realized in dance or other arts, we begin to have a glimpse of the way older adults may experience and find balance between the challenges, responsibilities, and pleasures they may come upon in older age.

Each person's story is important to hear. They reveal and portray common human concerns, strengths and weaknesses, as well as struggles and accomplishments. They allow us to dig deeper in our discovery of life's purpose and meaning. They reflect and reveal one's inspirations, and intuitively suggest ways of resolving problems and conflicts, making amends, and finding healing. Thus, as we further consider each person's life story, we realize the temporal dimensions of the person's past, present, and future. Each story reflects a timeline of the person's development, how they have become, and their vision of the future. We note too that throughout human history, stories have conveyed an expression of our creativity, and used to teach about and communicate essential understandings about our lives and the world in which we live, thereby passing this critical information on from one generation to the next. Indeed, we find the first examples of our use of stories and creative expression in the cave paintings, hieroglyphic inscriptions, oral traditions, and sacred texts of ancient communities throughout the world.[4] These early paintings, inscriptions, and oral and sacred expressions also reflect the earliest attempts to portray an understanding of our human nature. In later writings, both in the east and in the west, we find descriptions of how to understand and know ourselves.[5] In these texts we also find the roots of a mindset that seeks a deeper understanding of our human potential, similar to the existential and humanistic approaches in modern psychology.

We recognize too, the importance of our personal story as we share ideas about our everyday experiences with family and friends. As we relate our accomplishments, discuss insights and perspectives with others, we also gain a deeper understanding of the life we are living. Perhaps, in a most fundamental way, parents and grandparents are the first story tellers we meet. They are the conveyors of information about our families, our traditions, and our communities. Thus, the first stories we hear come from parents and grandparents, and later from the teachers and others we meet at school and through community and work experiences, also suggest to us a way of seeing and being in the world. They relate to us a philosophy about life, aid us in constructing a purposeful plan for our living, and make us aware of transcendental viewpoints, all of which may accompany us throughout our life journey.

"Aging is Not a Problem, Man"

When we review various research that portrays aging as a pathology and older adults as "sick," it motivates us to want to write about the complexities of growing older. In our view, growing older is not a disease requiring a cure, but rather a process in which we may discover deep personal insights, realize profound meaning as to the purpose of our life, and thus live in a more fulfilling manner. Of course, this is not to deny that we may encounter adverse and negative outcomes associated with growing older—and this presents the central complexity, paradox, and deeper process that we focus on in this book. The perspectives of Rollo May, Carl Rodgers, Irvin Yalom, and other humanistic and existential oriented thinkers convey a sense of this deeper process.[6] However, as the late sociologist Lars Tornstam suggests in his theory of Gerotranscendence, as younger people we are challenged by an age-associated "nearsightedness," that is, an inability to clearly understand and contemplate our later maturity and older age.[7] Moreover, even though we may have observed age-related biological and physical declines occurring in our family members, until it happens to us, we are rather limited in our understanding of what we might experience or be concerned with as we ascend to the end of the life-course. Indeed, it is difficult for any of us to foretell what our lives may be like in five or ten years. As we did when we were younger, we are likely to view the future rather egocentrically, from the perspective of how we are—perhaps relatively healthy, involved in our family life, work, and social obligations, and thus have a comparatively meager understanding of what might really occur as we age. We might think, for others at least, that later life will be a time of decline, disability, and illness. Certainly, what Tornstam infers is that as younger and midlife people we have not yet experienced the psychological landscape of later life and the challenges that our own aging may bring, and thus have scarce appreciation for what we have not yet lived. Further, as we look ahead to the future, we are likely to hold onto our optimistic biases and think all those "bad" things may not happen to us. We will enjoy life as we always did—and thus this is another facet of the paradox: "Aging is a not a problem, man" —until it is a problem.

Discovering the Arts of Living in Later Life

The dominant view of adult development and aging imposes a biomedical model to interpret the changes that occur as the person grows older. This model focuses on pathology, treatment, and cure. It is true that with advancing age there are gradual declines in physical capacities, sensory and cognitive abilities, and changes in psychological processes and social functioning, as well as increased risk for illness and disease. But these should not be seen to overshadow all the other positive and fulfilling aspects of our later maturity. In fact, much like we have experienced in earlier times of development, older age is a rather new adventure for each of us. Just like the first school picnic, getting your first job, or going on your first date, the experience of a new birthday, now in our 50s, or 60s, or 70s, or even 100s, is a new adventure—we haven't been here before! Furthermore, as we always adaptively seek to realize, despite the age-related changes that do occur, we are also likely to encounter moments of personal growth and new opportunities for an engaged and fulfilled life. Even as we grow older, we continue to learn, even if it may be diminished due to the challenges of illness or other neurological or health problems.

As one author of this book who has been involved with an intergenerational discussion forum for more than ten years notes, when there is free-exchange and conversation between older and younger people, it becomes clear that there are many insights and personal experiences that deepen our understanding of what it means to grow older. Insights into one's private accounts of aging that are often omitted or glossed over in the more technical and less personal scientific report. In their discussion, older and younger people share about their hopes for life and concerns about living. Their stories provide insight into unique as well as common experiences and tell us that older age and later life are not categories, but rather ongoing processes in human development. Importantly, an informed discussion about getting older, one that involves older people, reveals to us that many of the ideas we had

7

or what seemed so important early in our life, may not necessarily apply anymore when we are older. Moreover, because of these intergenerational exchanges, we have come to realize that through the telling and hearing of each person's life story, those of both younger and older persons, there is a great deal yet to learn!

We are more than the sum of our parts. Certainly, as we have seen in many instances after individuals recover from stroke or other brain injury, they may regain cognitive function and performance to near normal levels, despite rather radical neurological disruption. One of the authors through his research had the privilege to meet an older individual who performed at normal levels on tests of memory, despite having undergone rather drastic brain surgery earlier in life to treat epilepsy.[8] In another research encounter, the same author met with an older man who had moderate dementia of the Alzheimer's type. When asked if he would describe what he did the past weekend, he struggled to find the right words. He had difficulty putting his thoughts together to form an understandable sentence. It was difficult to comprehend what he was saying at first, but with careful listening and parsing together of story information, a connection was made. Pieced together, he indicated that he had attended a professional hockey game and had an exciting and enjoyable time with his family. As this understanding was relayed back to him, he smiled and beamed with happiness. In our brief exchange there was also a sharing of mutual support for the hometown team and mention of an article that appeared in the weekend sports section about the game. These examples suggest to us that even when there is rather moderate neurological loss or dementia, the neurons of our brains do not stop trying to make connections or stop "thinking." We also do not stop wanting to tell others about our lives, to express ourselves, and we do not stop learning. Rather life becomes more complex as we mature, often more interesting, and if we consider all the possibilities of what we might do next and how we might live, we find hints of how getting older can lead us in finding greater contentment and pleasure in life.

The Need to Create

One way we find contentment and pleasure is to live creatively. Further, through various artistic endeavors, we portray an authentic expression of our lives. As the philosopher Charles Taylor suggests, authenticity involves our creating, constructing, and discovering, while also seeking to be original and at times crossing over and operating beyond the boundaries of social convention.[9] Authenticity, Taylor claims, also requires movement to new points of view, self-definition, and self-realization. These later aspects suggest that in living authentically, we also experience change, transcending movement, and encounter new ways of being. Indeed, we are in constant movement from one state of existence to another. For example, we can see evidence of this transcendence when we recognize that who we were at age 18, is not necessarily the same person we are at age 60. In our transcendence into later life, we may also become more accepting of others and ourselves.[10] When we create and seek to discover and be original in our self-expression, we begin to live authentically. We transcend and move toward new ways of being. We recognize that it is alright to make mistakes, and if necessary, to start over again. In another way, we also create and recreate ourselves and, in this process, transcend and come to a new reality of who we are. Importantly, this process of creation and re-creation of self is set in motion, advanced, and revealed in our creative works, our arts, and our music. It is reflected in the stories we tell of our becoming, and in the stories told by others.

A Funny Thing Happened at the Music Festival

Upon attending a music festival recently that consisted of younger and "heritage" bands, it was interesting to note a relative age-related role-reversal of sorts, as the younger, first act warmed up the audience in anticipation of the older headline rock-star group. In contradiction to how later life is often described, i.e., as a time of decline, existential dread, and isolation, the younger warm-up band sang songs that echoed an angst and insecurity about life. While later, the older main-act group, along with added orchestral sections and replacement players filling-in for original band

9

members who had passed away long ago, sang songs of existential triumph and the celebration of life. It was a brilliant musical revery, exuding a sense of excitement about the great discoveries and experiences that await us in the next steps to be taken in one's development. Perhaps this role-reversal was intended to heighten the musical drama of the whole concert experience, or to provide the audience with a grand entrance into the musical magic and poetic allusion offered by the headline act. Regardless of intention, as put forth in Erik Erikson's psychosocial theory of development, the contrast in performances was reflective of the indecision many of us may have felt during adolescence or at the beginning of adulthood, and the powerful sense of generativity and integrity that may be experienced when we have been masterful in our living.[11] This realization stands in opposition to the various declines that are often so associated with growing older. Further, it underscores the importance of viewing later life beyond the eclipse of old-age stereotypes and depictions of later life portrayed in clinical and diagnostic medical terms that often suggest getting older to mean ever increasing limitation and ineptitude. Indeed, this music festival example bears evidence of how we might recognize the many possibilities and potentials of later life. Moreover, in this example we find the importance of seeking to explore and understand the personal experiences and concerns of midlife and older adults. Thus, looking beyond the inevitable physical changes and declines, and shifting patterns of social connections and involvements, we may discover new potentials and powers in older age.[12]

As we consider the possibilities of later life, we hope to reveal the many ways a person may continue in their creativity. Thus, as we begin to sketch out an approach that emphasizes ways in which we may grow in our personhood, we recognize the tensions and opportunities for the human family to grow in understanding and respect for all persons. Much like in previous ages, we recognize the possibility of moving forward in an enlightenment of reason and renaissance of thought, or regressing into a self-centered focus and diminishment of concern for other perspectives and ways of being. Yet as the renowned psychiatrist

Irvin Yalom has noted, from time to time, in considering how we explain and understand our world, we will need to construct a new paradigm. Thus, without equivocation, we too understand the need to re-examine, re-define and re-orient our system of explanation and understanding.[13] In order to see the potential of midlife and older adults in a realistic way, it behooves us to embrace an approach that depicts and describes the person in human terms, as an important member and contributor to family and community, regardless of changes in economic, physical, intellectual, or social status. Our goal then is to understand processes of maturation and growing older not strictly in the dynamics and features of disease, hospitalizations, and medical outcomes, but rather as opportunities when our living offers new and greater possibilities – where the maturity of later life is understood as a time that draws out from us our most advanced insights, creativity, and contributions.

The Deeper Concerns of Our Creativity

Our need to create reflects our unconscious drives for self-preservation, and the satisfaction of basic needs to belong and to love, to form family relationships, and to attain mastery in our living. But paradoxically, we also observe self-destructive instincts, risk-taking, aggressive behavior, murder, mayhem, and other acts that lead to our own destruction and that of others. Thus, the need to create reflects our attempt to address the most fundamental existential question of being and non-being, of existence and annihilation. Our creative expression is found in our thoughts, perceptions, and mental representations, in every memory and dream, and in our actions of becoming. Our creative expression is found in the line on the page that we draw, in the words we use when we speak and write, in the colors we choose to paint with, in the forms pressed into the clay we sculpt, and in our physical movements when we walk, jump, dance, and run. Indeed, throughout our life, in all our conscious and nonconscious activities, we are creative.

As children, most of us were involved in activities such as drawing and dancing, singing songs and making music, listening to, and telling stories, and a variety of other creative expressions.

Moreover, we *enjoyed* being creative! In many ways now in adulthood, we continue to enjoy these activities. Maybe it is because we use our creativity as a way of coping with the difficulties and challenges we meet in life. Certainly, our creative involvements are linked to wellness. As is well noted in various arts therapies, our creative expression serves as a way to overcome the problems we face. Indeed, through artistic and creative activities we can constructively channel our feelings of discontent and uneasiness and discover new ways to be in harmony with ourselves, with our families and others, and with our world. As Natalie Rogers suggests, when you find yourself in a place of dis-harmony, "You can dance your rage, paint your fear, or despair. Then several things happen: you discover how to find inner balance, inner peace... to have more compassion."[14] Fundamentally then, as we become involved in things like drawing and painting, photography and video-making, singing and playing music, dancing and physical movement arts, quilting and knitting, composing stories and poems, dramatic expression and storytelling, or immersed in listening, reading, and attending creative exhibits and performances, we discover new approaches and ways of responding to the challenges we face and the world in which we live. Our creativity connects us to the most vital aspects of what it means to be human. Our artistic and creative practices refresh and revitalize us. Through them we re-frame our concerns and are directed in the next steps of our becoming. Our artistic and creative endeavors transmit an expression of our hopes for, and insights into, and understandings of the life that we live and share with others.

Walt Whitman: A Poet's Self-Discovery and Celebration in Later Life

As Walt Whitman expresses, in older age we may discover new perspectives, and a wider and deeper understanding of life. Born in Huntington, New York, in 1819, and raised in Brooklyn, as a young man Whitman worked at many jobs in the printing and newspaper industry, beginning a very prolific career as a writer and poet.[15] Yet, his work, even until the end of his life, did not find wide acceptance, and thus he briefly tried teaching, served as a volunteer nurse in army hospitals during the American Civil War, was a clerk with the U.S. Interior Department, and eventually gaining later success with his writing, settled on being a poet. Receiving greater acclaim and recognition posthumously than he did while he lived, Whitman's poetry provides insight into the historic and sociocultural moment in which he lived, as well as his self-reflections on maturing and growing older. Further, despite suffering a series of strokes that caused paralysis and depression in his 50s, Whitman continued to rejoice in the moment, expressing the intuitions and wonder of later life.[16] As remarked by a peer of his time, Canadian psychiatrist Dr. Richard M. Bucke, much like the insights conveyed by such great figures as Socrates, Buddha, Jesus, and Mohammed, Whitman's prose and poetry reflects a cosmic consciousness, or mystical illumination and expression that conveys a universal truth about our human experience.[17] Thus, throughout Whitman's poetry, we sense the expression of later life's magical and mystical moments that can only be found through processes of self-reflection. In poems such as "Twilight" and "Memories," he notes the contrast as well as connection between times of youth and older age, and suggests that in the moment of our twilight we may discover an oblivion and revelry. In the poems, "To Get the Final Lilt of Songs," "Continuities," and "Thanks in Old Age," Whitman recognizes that "shifting spheres," or changes in our appearances or situations, should not distract us from finding insight and joy in the new discovery that avails itself through the continuing quest to find meaning in our lives.

The Paradoxes of Aging

We are always on a path of self-discovery. In our living and continuing development, the deeply reflective Whitman suggests we still have questions to ask and ideas to understand; questions of personal identity and of how we may re-make ourselves. We see in Whitman's poem "Queries to my Seventieth Year," that one of the paradoxes of aging is the existential duality of getting older: Will I yet find life and wonder in my living, or will I experience the darkness of my dying as I encounter age-related physical and mental declines?[18] As we move through life, we too will contemplate the duality of our existence. Reflective of our basic humanity, this duality—this paradox—is illustrated in the contrasts of physical decline but possible spiritual awakening, sense of belonging and isolation, fulfillment and loss, and satisfaction and struggle. This duality is also found in our artistic expression vis a vis getting older, in that we can be our most creative in older age, but also begin to witness serious decline in our abilities to create the art we so much enjoy. How can we begin then to understand this paradox, this duality of our being? One way we propose is to realize the continued need for artistic expression as we grow older, and the ways of personal discovery and fulfilled living both our creativity and aging offer.

Another paradox of aging involves the concept of "successful aging." The notion of "successful aging," as part of one's process of becoming, ignores that not all of us age "successfully," or in the same way. To present one without the other deludes us into thinking that setbacks, ill-health, or failures separate us from other human beings, and leads us to believe that we are unique in our ability not to be able to rise above our failings. Therefore, "successful aging" seems too narrow, too westernized, and too static of a concept. It expresses that good health, economic security, social and cultural well-being are the benchmarks of aging well, but do not address declines in our physical prowess and health, cognitive, interpersonal and social changes, and ultimately death that awaits us at the end of our life. In this instance, the narrowness and simplicity of the term omits the more complex reality that we all face as we grow older. One resolution to this paradox, as Socrates had comparably noted, is to recognize the many dimensions of our lives and the greater complexity of our experience as we get older. When we do this, we may also realize that in all those moments where we have had to re-define ourselves due to physical or cognitive limitations, or adjust when social relationships change or end, or revise our philosophy of living when we encountered existential challenges, that we also discovered and were led onto pathways where we found a more complete and more fulfilling way of living.

A related paradox highlights the distinction between specific qualities or features of life and the wholeness of the person. Specific qualities or features might be illustrated by goals we achieve, or our awards or personal accomplishments, or other identified benchmarks such as starting a career or raising a family. Focusing on wholeness, however, goes beyond these specific features to an assessment of one's life as a totality. Both perspectives are important, yet neither completely informs us about the person or how one might construct knowledge about the human condition. For example, it sounds rather quixotic when we hear someone say, "Gee, I feel young in lots of ways, even though this birthday I am another year older!" The argument to consider here is that both the whole and the smaller features or aspects of the person and their life as they get older, are one. This resolution inferring wholeness is characteristic of a more universal orientation, one that moves past the impediments of scientific paradigms, cultural settings, or social stratifications. Indeed, it embraces a humanistic, experiential orientation. This wholeness approach includes and considers all aspects of what it means to be human and to become as we continue into later life.

Another paradox involves how we construct meaning, and how we come to "know" things. The question is how does this epistemology driven not only by scientific or empirical methods, but also by one's creative expressions such as poems, stories, artwork, and music provide us with a realistic and truthful interpretation of later life? Certainly, how we come to know things and construct meaning is intertwined within the sciences and the arts. We know that both the specific empirical and the more creative and philosophical approaches are related, thus we propose that through a resolution that recognizes the equal importance of the two, we can embrace a more complete picture of aging.

We can begin to reason about and to resolve these paradoxes in two ways. The first is that we live in a liminal space of existence. In other words, that our living involves transitions. The second way is that the apparent duality of our living is not an either-or experience, but one in which contrasting opposites occur simultaneously.

15

Liminal Space

Liminal space is considered to represent a transition, a rite of passage, a change from one state to another. It can contain good and bad elements. For example, we can think of living along with the certainty that one day we will die. Often this liminal space is filled with anxiety, ambiguity, and tension. In medicine, we can think of liminal space for organ transplantation. Here the patient is in the role of not only a sick person, but also a post-transplant person, and reflecting on the concepts of normality in what defines being healthy. In end stage diseases such as cancer or Alzheimer's disease, the liminal space is one of moving from a sick role to a dying role, or from life to death. Thus, embracing the concept of liminal space allows us to approach our paradoxes. We can discard outdated concepts of aging and move toward an understanding of the complexities of our existence—that we are in the here and now, but also moving toward the future—to a different state. This understanding provides us with a way toward wholeness, to deeper appreciation of our experiences, and a life filled with profound meaning.

Concepts of Duality Occur Simultaneously

We tend to believe that much of our living involves a duality of existence. We can express our life in dichotomous terms such as happiness-sadness, grief-joy, ascent-decent and so on. This perspective of duality is well-grounded in many Eastern philosophical approaches. For example, the concept of Yin and Yang in Chinese philosophy represent a duality. Yin contains female aspects of the universe, whereas Yang represents male aspects. Although they are contrasts, it is important to note that they also move beyond duality. That is, they also complement one another in that each contains an aspect of the other. The wholeness or oneness of Yin and Yang are key in Traditional Chinese Medicine, with the basis being that when the forces of Yin and Yang are out of balance, ill health occurs.

Thus, we propose that the idea of existence as a duality is something of an illusion that implies that these states are categorical and at odds with each other. This categorical distinction of duality is primarily a Western approach. Whereas we take a more Eastern approach to duality and to aging. We offer that to resolve the paradoxes established earlier is to understand that these dualities occur simultaneously, thus providing us a way to contemplate getting older, achieving wholeness, and assigning meaning to our lives. The key is to understand the simultaneous existence of opposites, and as Carl Jung proposed, to ultimately achieve "liberation from opposites," and to be able to express opposites as if they were one and the same "breath."[19] When we recognize this oneness, we are able to move beyond the current zeitgeist of the biomedical model of aging, and begin to experience and journey into the deeper and more profound psychology of later life.

Certainly, our lives are in transition, we exist in a liminal space, but also in one of simultaneous contrasts. In effect, we are always in the where-we-were of our lives, the where-we-are-now, and the where-we-will-be. But again, the key is to understand that the where-we-were, and the where-we-are-now still exist at the same time! Although the past can be dimmed by time and distorted or forgotten from memory, it still represents a part of our existence that somehow does not magically become "boxed" away or forgotten, but exists at the same time as our present experience. Moreover, our thoughts of the future, although more ephemeral, are intertwined with our past and present experiences. Thus, as we come to the realization that although our life experiences are unique to us as a person, they also reflect a universality to our existence as a species, one that we all share. From this perspective, we can see the lives of each person, without limitation or restrictions, as equally valuable and worthy of our appreciation and respect. It is by being creative, through our involvement with the arts, that we connect with and understand our commonality with others, and in turn the process of getting older more completely. We can move beyond the concepts of duality, beyond an us versus them thinking and either-or mentalities, and boldly face the challenges that we will meet and thus live more authentically.

This book presents stories of people. Some of the stories are about famous people, but many come from people who are not famous. Some of the stories were gathered through interviews for this book, other stories come from our allied and supplemental research, teaching practices, and conversations with friends, family, and associates. Following a narrative approach that explores existential concerns, we use an interviewing method that does not incorporate a set order of questions, but rather focuses on the person's creative interests, experiences, insights, and outlook on life. Each person's story is important, and we thank those who, through their kind permission, have allowed us to tell their stories. Their accounts reference common struggles and concerns we all face, and suggest how that through our creative expression and involvement in such endeavors as prose writing, needle-work, music-making, painting, carving, sculpture, dance, and gardening, to name a few, we may transcend to a greater and more fulfilling way of life.

Upon entering the nature preserve, hiking along a well-traveled path, there were things to be seen that I hadn't noticed before – new plants and blooming flowers; trees and foliage whose branches reached out in new directions. From one season to the next there occurs a noticeable change in the preserve. But treasuring nature's beauty this day, I sensed I had changed too. In a way, I felt I had become more receptive to the new blooms and expanding foliage, and more appreciative of the warmth of the glowing sunshine that beamed through the tree canopy. An ancient understanding that still informs contemporary psychology is that "we don't see the world as it is, we see the world as we *are*." So, what had changed in me?

When we consider how we may grow and become, we recognize the various factors that shape and direct our development throughout the life-course, as well as the nurturing assistance of caregivers and others that help us in overcoming the many challenges we encounter along the way. As the poem, "Children Learn What They Live" by Dorothy Law Nolte suggests, if we are brought up in an environment that is deriding and filled with put-downs, with threats of violence to oneself or family, without support from parents and the broader social community, we are likely to grow up with an attitude that at times is condemning, demeaning, and hostile towards others.[1] We are also likely to continue cycles of miscommunication and violence in family relations, and exhibit disrespect, division, and inequality within our communities. In comparison, if we are brought up in an environment where we feel loved, have the positive support of parents, family, and community, and are encouraged in our choices and next steps in development as a person, we are more likely to become loving, supportive, and nurturing toward ourselves and others. Even in later life, we may reflect on the various aspects of the environments in which we have grown up. We may at times express social stereotypes, biases, and prejudices, or in contrast, attitudes of mutual respect and acceptance that we have been taught. Most of us remember when someone was mean to us, and perhaps also know about our tendencies to react toward others in a similar manner; or remember when we had received special assistance with or backing for the life-choices we made, and our ongoing hope to also respond toward others with an attitude of acceptance and support. For many of us, we realize too that we have not quite mastered all the things we hope to learn in life. Not to mention finding a deeper understanding of how our earlier experiences shaped the way we are now, as we revise and tell our life stories at midlife or in older age.

Indeed, it is not easy work, as the great author, educator, and heroine of self-discovery Helen Keller recognized beginning her autobiography:

> It is with a kind of fear that I begin to write the history of my life. I have… a superstitious hesitation in lifting the veil that clings about my childhood like a golden mist. The task of writing an autobiography is a difficult one… many of the joys and sorrows of childhood have lost their poignancy; and many incidents of vital importance in my early education have been forgotten in the excitement of great discoveries.[2]

An exceptional person and inspiring figure throughout her life, Helen Keller was stricken with an illness resulting in a brain fever (now thought to be caused by scarlet fever or meningitis) at 19 months of age. As a result, she became blind and deaf, and faced immense challenges throughout life. However, possessing an indomitable life spirit, and with the help of her teacher Anne Sullivan, she learned finger spelling that allowed her to communicate. Later, Helen learned to speak under the tutelage of Sarah Fuller of the Horace Mann School for the Deaf and attended Radcliffe College where she graduated cum laude. Among her many accomplishments, she wrote fourteen books and more than 475 speeches and essays, and co-founded the American Civil Liberties Union in 1920.[3] Helen Keller was also a world-renowned advocate for the prevention of blindness and for the creation of education and job-placement programs to assist people with disabilities. Thus, as we consider life stories, and those as exceptional as that of Helen Keller's, we understand that in many ways we are different in later life than we were earlier in our development, and through this understanding come to new insights and discoveries that direct how we perceive, think about, and interact in our present world.

In this chapter we will begin to explore life-stories and describe ways we may discover new patterns in our unfolding personal history, and by doing so, we lift the veil revealing a new light of understanding that may direct us onto new pathways and ways of being. We will also note the deeper aspects of our psychology expressed in stories and conclude by discussing individuals who may inspire us in our lives.

Discovery in Self-Reflection

Self-reflection is a perspective taking process that extends to the earliest times in human history. Attempts to know oneself were prescribed by the ancient Greeks as a fundamental method to understand how to be happy and live in harmony with others. In our contemporary world, this introspection, or looking inward and evaluating our feelings and the logical truth of our thoughts, is a key pursuit in psychoanalysis and cognitive-emotive behavior therapies. It is in these processes of looking inward that we find insight into how we construct our inner world, how we make decisions, and how we overcome challenges that occur in life. As we move through and transcend the life-course, however, we often understand our life experiences in different ways. For example, by the time we enter adulthood, life may seem to have become so regular that we feel many everyday experiences are rather passé. Sometimes too, we may have felt that what we knew so well is no longer relevant, or somehow incorrect as we consider new discoveries or different points of view. We may have experienced times of disillusionment, of moving beyond fantasy into a more appropriate realism, or in sensing an enlightenment and advancement in our thinking. Indeed, such new discovery is conveyed in the saying often attributed to humorist and writer

Samuel Clemens (Mark Twain): "When I was a boy of 14, my father was so ignorant I could hardly stand to have the old man around. But when I got to be 21, I was astonished at how much the old man had learned in seven years."

Certainly, by one's 40th or 50th birthday, there has been a lot of living that has occurred, and a lot of learning too. We have recognized physical changes that affect how youthful and attractive we may look, as well as our strength and stamina to run and jump and play sports like we did earlier in life. But when considering emotional and intellectual resources, and the mastery of various practical skills and abilities, the person at midlife may still be yet far-off from the peak expression of their talents and creativity. Indeed, at midlife we might realize, like the hiker in the nature preserve noted above, that there are many new things to look forward to, many new buds and blossoms along life's path yet to appreciate. We may seek a deeper understanding of ourselves, and express a greater appreciation for the meaningful interactions we might have with intimate others, children, and older parents. Further, we may sense a deeper enjoyment in our job and work routines, and perhaps even the rather mundane aspects of our living. In later life too, at times we may find that despite nagging physical complaints or challenging illness and health crises, that we have a new freedom in our self-expression, and a deeper understanding of what our life means. Through our self-reflections we may find a deeper insight into who we are, what we are about, and new inspiration to be creative and to share the many gifts we have with those around us.

The "Telling" of Our Life Story

As established in oral history projects such as Studs Terkel's *Working*, Bernice Neugarten's *The Meanings of Age*, and Dave Isay's *StoryCorps Project*, a person's story is a window into their deepest concerns and experiences of living.[4] Our stories portray the interests and apprehensions that shape our living, from the very earliest times in development to the present moment and provide a vantage point from which to consider the future. Moreover, our stories elucidate psychosocial, cultural, historic, and generational influences on how we become, and thus provide a key method to understand processes of adult development and aging.[5] Therefore, apart from the great insights the clinical and experimental sciences provide in explaining human behavior, our stories are a rich resource that help us to understand the more delicate, intricate, and masked aspects of our human nature.

As we have suggested above, the contexts in which we live and the challenges we face affect how we become. For our personal development, context and challenge are like the tempering of iron-based metal, that through the great heating and cooling that follows, a steel of great strength may be forged. Thus, when we consider our life stories, we also recognize the circumstances and experiences of living which have placed great pressures on us and enhanced our personal strengths. Indeed, one's personal history provides insight into processes of maturation and change, of particular crises and times of celebration, and ways of coping as one enters the second half of the life course. In the collection of these life stories, beyond the elaboration on risk for disease, medical classifications, and diagnostic labels of aging, we find great insight into and profound explanation of the experiences of midlife and older age. And it is correct to say, "collection of life stories," because there are many chapters and sub-plots, many key exchanges within the dialogue between characters, and a variety of descriptions of our sensory experiences in the unfolding of one's life. Sometimes the stories express an elation—a new time of life or new achievement attained, and the happiness felt. At other moments they might express a free-falling freedom, a movement beyond past inhibitions or disillusionments. This notion of "free-fall" in physics refers to movement by gravitational pull. Implied as a psychological status, it might refer to the loss of control when someone falls in love, or as one breaks free from a quagmire of constraining emotions and negative facets of self-identity.

Furthermore, with an increase in the world-wide ageing population, being aware of the older person's life story has been important for interpreting their quality of life and in providing appropriate health care. As Karen Van Leeuwen and colleagues have emphasized, when seeking to understand the health and well-

23

being of older people, it is important to know what the person believes contributes to a quality of life, and what they consider important in their healthcare.[6] For healthcare providers, knowing about the older person's life story results in increased personalized communication, and offers opportunities for the caregiver to provide an enhanced quality of care.[7] For the older adult too, there is a sense that they are being heard, and that their life and personal concerns matter. We will go more in-depth about how our life story may be used therapeutically in the next chapter, but let's look closer at what we find in these stories.

Life Story: Contexts, Common Plots, and Characteristic Roles

We have always told a story about ourselves. A life story conveys our personal history—our experiences, relationships, hopes, defeats, and achievements. Our stories provide the context for our life. It tells others who we are. If you think back, you might remember an early time in preschool or elementary grades when you told a classmate about where you lived, what your parents did for a living, and what things you did for fun, and pastimes you liked best. That early story changed as you advanced in school, and included features about what you hoped to do when you became older. By late adolescence and early adulthood our life story was already well elaborated, and often described our special talents, experiences, and dreams for the future. That early adulthood story also likely contained private episodes, parts about yourself that you did not want to make public and preferred to be kept confidential.

We could only imagine in childhood what adulthood and older age might be like. You might also remember hearing the stories of parents and grandparents. Recalling those family stories, we identify historic or economic influences that may have limited opportunities for educational and specialized training, or placed special demands on the individual to work to help their family or to serve their country. For example, many of us have heard stories about grandfathers who entered the workforce after completing a schooling that taught the basic necessities of reading, writing, and arithmetic, or quit high school or college because they enlisted or were drafted into the armed services. Or of grandmothers who had the opportunity to attend college but only graduated with their high-school diploma before getting married, starting, and caring for a family, or going to work. While these types of stories may seem to reflect a distant past, they also describe contextual features of the place and historic moment in which the person lived that become central features of one's life story.

When we look more closely at stories and the people involved, we are also likely to find other common features. In a critical examination of the stories that make up classic myths, novels, plays, movies, and television soap-operas, and the one's in which we talk about ourselves, Christopher Booker suggests there are seven basic plots and a recurring cast of heroes-heroines, villains, and supporting characters.[8] Further, he suggests we have a psychological need to create and tell stories as a way of expressing our human nature and to find meaning and purpose in life. To be sure, we are commentators on life, announcing our hopes and concerns, as well as the objects of our desires and our rationale for seeking them—hoping to provide a narrative that will provide insight into and solution for our existential concerns.

Thus, it is not surprising then to recognize the seven basic plots that we give ear to, and often reference as we tell about ourselves or others, include, firstly, "fighting the monster." To vanquish the monster, we must overcome some great external or internal foe, or an evil outside or inside of us, and if we are victorious, we may achieve a sense of self-virtue or come to a new self-realization. The second common plot is a "rags to riches" story. Here we are set against a bad fate and must overcome impossible odds to achieve a happy ending. The story plot may involve not only exterior challenges, but again a mastery of our will to persevere, to hope, to overcome, even when it may seem impossible. Many of the plots may over-lap somewhat, so other common types of storylines put forth by Booker that describe "a quest" and "a voyage and return," seem to do this. These plots refer to the testing and growth of the self, but importantly a metamorphosis and transformation of being that occurs from encountering extreme challenges. The fifth and sixth common plots proposed by Booker are "comedy" and "tragedy." Most of us wish to seek out fun and happy moments for our lives—making jest about the mundane as well as the more difficult and tragic aspects of living. But again, like the quest and voyage plots, these storylines allow us to see ourselves in serious and not so serious ways, and inform us on how to discover deeper meaning about our lives. The seventh and final common plot suggested by Booker is "rebirth," and refers again to transformation and new insight into how we may imagine our being. What is interesting to note is that we are all likely to live out these plots in some manner or other in the dramatic scenes of our life. We will fight to defeat a monster, seek to attain a happy ending, and take on challenges of great quests and voyages from which we return changed. We will live a life with moments deserving of comic relief and at times imperiled with great tragedy, and, as we contemplate our birth and death, we may pray for and hope to experience rebirth.

While we may consciously script out the scenes of our life, we can only imagine and act out these various plots through the expression of our deeper psychology. Thus, when we cast the actors and roles of each plot, we also reveal unconscious motives and archetypal dimensions of our self. Indeed, as Carl Jung and other theorists of his school have suggested, when we look at the cast of characters in our dreams and in our life-stories, we often find the same actors: The Hero and Heroine, the Savior, the Protector, and the Guardian. Further, we also come upon other archetypal representations found within the collective unconscious that are comforting and enlightening: The Caring Father or Loving Mother figures, the Sage, Mentor, and Everyman. As Jung further notes, there is an opposite side too, one that reflects the primitive Shadow aspects of our psychology. These figures are representative of more primitive facets of our human nature, and usually reflect our impulses for aggression and sensual gratifications. Thus, the Villain, Siren, or Trickster are common archetypes that often fill out the rest of our cast. Jung suggested there may be many different archetypal images, but he was most interested in the private, inner Self, that directs the outward facing Persona we project publicly, as well as the dynamic Anima/Animus, and the dark and largely instinctive, unknown, and often uncontrollable Shadow.

When we recount our life story and talk about our families then, we often tell stories that reveal common themes and archetypal characteristics. Undeniably, our personal stories describe our activities, challenges, culture, and the expectations we hold for ourselves. Talking about our families is also a way of telling others about ourselves, and the challenges and gifts that families provide. For example, a wonderful father, always caring and interested, might also be the same person who was overbearing, or drank too much at family reunions, or blew up easily if things did not work out as planned. In many ways then, our personal and family stories begin to explain what we value and hold sacred in life; why we may react or behave in a particular way; why we made certain life-choices or followed a path of our own making. In sharing our deepest intimacies, our storytelling also aids us in forming caring friendships and developing strong social bonds with others. Especially in later life, we might savor the opportunity to have a discussion at mealtime with family members, to share about and review the day's events, and to consider challenges, express hopes, and revel in the celebration of the day.

A Later life Paradox: No Role Models?

We often believe that we are the main character in life's play and agent of our own action. However, at other times, we may feel that we no longer control events, but that events now control us. In a related way, the dramatic plot can be complex, and the significance of particular characters rather dynamic and important, or fleeting and seemingly non-existent in another person's storytelling. For example, there is an interesting phenomenon called the Spotlight Effect that illustrates the egocentric bias in our perceptions of importance to others, and how much attention people really pay to us. Researchers who investigated this effect, asked people to wear a T-shirt in the presence of others that would "potentially" draw attention to them. In one interesting study, participants were asked to wear a T-shirt with a big picture of Barry Manilow, the well-known singer and songwriter, on the front. Those who wore the shirt later reported that they felt that everyone was looking at them and that they were put in the "spotlight" and became the center of attention. However, when other people in the room were asked if they recalled seeing someone wearing something odd, most reported to have seen nothing unusual![9] Thus, while we most often play the central role in our stories, sometimes we may not be cast as an important or even recognizable character in the story of others.

Although we wish to highlight the arts as an avenue to celebration in later life, not everyone may perceive the experiences of getting older or the transitions into later life in a positive way. For example, in poignant conversations with older professors of life-span development who were close to, or already in retirement, it was puzzling and somewhat concerning to note their great discontent and dispiritedness about later life, and hear some of them say, "There are no role models for me in old age!" "There is no one to look to—no one to draw inspiration from!" At first blush, it is hard to know what to make of these statements. Maybe they were correct—in later life there is no positive example to follow, no one to inspire us to meet the challenges of later life or motivate us to write our own epic stories. Or worse, that in older age we no longer matter, that our lives no longer have meaning, that we have nothing to offer to others. But as we do not want to write off their remarks to a despair or discontent about older age, we propose that they importantly tell us something profound. Such remarks convey something we will confront at some point in our lives: being in a crisis, at a point of transition, where one may not know how to move forward into the next stage of life. It may also reflect a limited awareness or outlook, that in comparison to one's present circumstances, is based on the achievements and standards of an earlier time in life. This earlier way of seeing ourselves may narrow our vision for what is possible in the future. In addition, as expressed in the invincible spirit and life of Helen Keller, our "vision" of the future is an inner reality of the person, and closely associated with how the person hopes to see themselves living in the world. Thus, like in earlier times of development, in later life we will also adaptively seek to overcome challenges, and discover a personal sense of integrity, an inner resource, that empowers us to live confidently and compose the next chapters in the story of our life.

Furthermore, while role models have been noted as an important influence on the young person in forming their identity and striving to reach their greatest potential, there is a paucity of research on role models in older age groups. The few studies involving midlife and older adults often narrowly define the role model construct as one's commitment to and satisfaction derived from work, or healthy aging, or successful aging.[10] These studies suggest that there may be both positive and negative role models in later life. That is, there exists an assortment of positive characteristics (e.g., commitment to work, success in career, active in exercise routines, in good health and high cognitive functioning) and negative characteristics (e.g., use of alcohol or smoking, cognitive or physical declines), that, respectively, we might hope to embrace and emulate, or seek to steer clear of and avoid. Although, while role models can often include family members (e.g., parents, grandparents, extended family members), one study reported that 15 percent of the sample did not name a "successful aging" role model. Perhaps this lack of role models in later life is due to the undesirable beliefs we may hold about aging or how we view older people. Maybe it stems from an anxiety about getting older. It may result from our sense of failure to attain the goals of successful aging: personal control and autonomy, above average social engagement, almost perfect health, or substantial wealth. In some way we may believe that we do not measure up to the standards that we, society, and others set for ourselves.

We propose an alternative view to move us past these negative self-reflections and toward a path of renewal and hope. This view is that our role models do not have to be those who demonstrate feats of superhuman strength or those that have overcome insurmountable odds. Our role models should probably not be based on the "successful aging trifecta" of great wealth, excellent health, and impassioned social involvements. In many ways, our lives are filled with struggles that are ongoing and often the heroic stance is to endure. Perhaps in our endurance others can take inspiration from us, and, importantly, we may find an inner strength to go on. At any time in life, our role models can be just regular, everyday people. Maybe it is a single mom who raises a teenage son and two younger daughters, meeting the demands of parenting and family life while working two jobs. Or a grandpa and grandma who serve as guardians, raising a grandchild because their son or daughter cannot. As we broaden our consideration of who might serve as a role model, perhaps it is someone like Malala Yousafzai, advocate for the rights of women and girls and youngest Nobel Prize laureate, or Sir David Attenborough, broadcaster, writer, naturalist, and biologist. Respectively younger and older persons, who through their championing of social justice and environmental concerns, have raised awareness and inspired others to also serve as guardians of human rights and protectors of the earth. Moreover, given the wealth of experience acquired as we practice our professions, mature and grow older, sharing our wisdom and insights is an important role for each of us. Thus, in later life we may model our ethical values and moral approach to life as we provide assistance and support to younger people as they take on life's many challenges.

Helen Keller: An Epitome of Creativity and Life Celebration

As we contemplate the personal courage we need to meet and overcome a wide variety of life challenges, we again return to the story of Helen Keller. Despite being blind and deaf, Helen Keller lived very vibrantly, creatively expressing her great optimism for living. Active in her advocacy for people with disabilities, she was an inspiration and role model to people throughout the world. In her life she travelled to all continents except Antarctica, interacting and corresponding with world leaders, leading scientists, celebrities, and many admiring fans and supporters. Throughout her 70s, she continued to travel the world advocating for people with disabilities and social justice causes. She had a stroke at 81 years of age which caused her to limit her public outings but continued in her very positive outlook on life. Thus, she truly may be proclaimed as a heroine of self-discovery, and an epitome of creativity and celebration of life. In her essay, *Optimism*, she relates a personal story that describes her deeply reflective and resilient nature, and her choice to always frame the challenges of living in a positive way:

> Most people measure their happiness in terms of physical pleasure and material possession… If happiness is to be so measured, I who cannot hear or see have every reason to sit in a corner with folded hands and weep. If I am happy in spite of my deprivations, if my happiness is so deep that it is a faith, so thoughtful that it becomes a philosophy of life, — if, in short, I am an optimist, my testimony to the creed of optimism is worth hearing.[11]

* * *

In a "Scrapbook of Hellen Keller and the Blind" created by Rebecca Mack, there contains a newspaper clipping from the Sunbury, Pennsylvania's *Daily Item*, entitled, "Confidently Climb the Stair." This brief article once again reveals Helen Keller's essence, her unconquerable nature and optimistic attitude, and gives us insight into how we might also view getting older and later life. As the article relates, when asked by a high school student about her approach to older age, she responded saying she views aging, much like blindness, as an individual problem—everyone will come to experience its uplifting high points, and its ominous low points. In conveying her story, Helen Keller relates her belief that with advancing age comes the greatest harvest of happiness, and just as true sight and hearing comes from within, not from without, so will the discovering of new aspects of the person and our enthusiasm for and celebration in later life. We share below excerpts from the story published May 3, 1950, in the newspaper, *Daily Item:*

Confidently Climb the Stair

You are the first person who has asked me pointblank that question. I cannot help smiling—I who have declared these many years that there is no age to the spirit. Age seems to me only another physical handicap, and it excites no dread in my mind—I who have lived so triumphantly with my limitations.

Once I had a dear friend of 80 who said she enjoyed life more at that age than she had at 25. Never count how many years you have, this friend would say, but how many interests. Then and there I resolved to cherish an inextinguishable flame of youth. All my life I have tried to avoid ruts, such as doing things my ancestors did before me, or leaning on the crutches of other people's opinions, or losing my childhood sense of wonderment. I am glad I still have a vivid curiosity about the world I live in. Now, in answer to your question: I suppose that age, like blindness, is an individual problem. Everybody discovers its roseate mountain peaks, its gloomy depths, according to his or her temperament. It is natural for me to believe that the richest harvest of happiness comes with age as to believe that true sight and hearing are within, not without. Confidently I climb the broad stairway that love, and faith have built, to the heights where I shall look out upon other, higher peaks beyond. For there is always something better farther on. [12]

Being Creative in How We Become

Writing many books, essays, and speeches, and active in her advocacy for people with disabilities, Helen Keller continues to serve as a wonderful model for how we might live in later life. Her great enthusiasm and spirit of overcoming reflects what is possible in our living. Such a creative and optimistic outlook is also noted in a more recent contemporary figure, Amanda Gorman, the youngest Inaugural Poet of the United States. Ms. Gorman through her poetry and human rights advocacy, much Like Helen Keller, also suggests how we may "climb" in our work against the oppression and marginalization of any person. Certainly, it will require us to be creative and sensitive in our self-reflection, to consider actions that we may take to make the world a better place. This is even more challenging as we realize the changes that must occur within ourselves—in the re-adjustment of our values, attitudes, intentions, and willingness to respect and treat all persons and communities equally. The verses of Ms. Gorman's Inauguration poem "The Hill We Climb" directs us to be brave in our work for every person's freedom – for each person's respectful, compassionate, and equitable treatment– and in our own process of becoming.[13] To live a joyful and fulfilled later life, we must create a story that leads to our transformation. So that the answer to "how have we changed?" is plainly shown in how we have become.

Our life stories reflect our earliest experiences and influences. As the great playwright and poet William Shakespeare so keenly observed, and announces in *King Henry IV* through the character The Earl of Warwick: there is a history in each person's life; a story of how they are known and how one may know themselves, which orients and directs the many steps a person will take throughout their life journey.[1] Similarly, in the play, *The Tempest*, Shakespeare again dramatically suggests how our history influences our future, as the character Antonio announces, "What's past is prologue."[2] Thus, for good or bad, in our earliest life experiences a groundwork is set for the things that may occur later in life. It might be what our parents did for a living and the way they created a family life, our cultural perspective or faith tradition, or family's history of and risk for illness. In this chapter we will continue to consider the artful ways we go about talking about ourselves and addressing our existential concerns, and how family stories may influence our present living. We will also note the therapeutic benefits of telling our life story. In a sense, how the telling of our life story may enhance our living, help us to slay the dragons of our past, and find our current daily experiences as moments of celebration.

Stories Connect Us

Stories connect us with one another and express our communally shared values and creeds. In them we grasp the threads of our past and reveal the evolving social structures and psychological aspects of our current living. Our stories often seek to address and resolve the existential uncertainties of death, personal freedom, isolation, and meaninglessness; matters of such profound and ultimate concern, according to psychotherapist Irvin Yalom, that all people encounter and may struggle with in life.[3] So it is not surprising that our stories are key to the implementation of a patient-centered style of care, and in facilitating the processes of life-review and reminiscence in later life.[4]

Working as college professors of psychology, both in our teaching and research we have had the very good fortune to encounter people at all points along the life-course and to learn of their life. In our conversations with them, whether young, midlife, or older adult, we have become cognizant of the common threads that draw into focus the existential enquiries posed since ancient times: How do I understand my origin? How might I understand or overcome my past? How can I be happy? What will the future be like? Reflectively, these concerns are like the tidal forces of the sea. They direct our thinking, feeling, and acting, and are communicated in one's creative works and life's endeavors.[5] As personality psychologist Dan McAdams has noted, our personal story is created early in development and revised throughout the life course.[6] It contains various narrative tones, expressing emotions such as anger, disgust, fear, happiness, surprise, and sadness, and communicate the beliefs, values, and motives that direct our actions and ways of viewing ourselves and the world. Our stories also contain points of beginning, periods of enduring, points of transition and places of ending, and convey our legacy and how we and others may begin anew. Importantly, as we tell our life story, we describe our families and community, and provide a basic portrayal of the contexts in which we have grown up and live.

Our Family's Past Influences the Present and Future

Our lives are connected to our parents and to all our family lineage. Thus, it is not uncommon as we begin to tell our life story that we refer to our parents and members of our family from generations past. In doing so, we recognize that our identity is anchored in and arises from our family and communal history. Further, in our artful storytelling we undertake a personal journey of self-discovery, distinguishing our cultural background as well as our relatedness to and an identification with our ancestors.[7] Indeed, as writer and literary scholar Patrick Colm Hogan suggests, when we tell of or hear about the lives of our family and community, we empathetically establish and discern the universal story-plots of sacrifice, heroism, romantic love, and re-imagine and sense a sharing of common experiences and feelings.[8]

Examples of this empathic involvement is found in the following stories shared by two retired teachers, Ben Cruz-Uribe and Eileen Johnson. Each offers the back-story about members of the person's family, and tells of origin events that are shared and carried with the storyteller now. Further, in their storytelling, we find recognizable plots involving trials and tribulations, personal duty and sacrifice, advantages and disadvantages, and romantic yearnings as we hear of the noble characteristics and intrepid nature of family members from generations past. In their narrative accounts, as Ben and Eileen herald the special qualities of the stories' protagonists, they also tell us of themselves. In doing so, they tacitly reveal the familial and cultural bonds they share with the actors, and deep moral aspects of the story which have inspired them and continue to shape their personhood.

Ben Cruz-Uribe: Stories of Ancestors

Constructed from personal observations, letters, and other historical artifacts, Ben Cruz-Uribe tells the following stories:

> The stories that I will share are of my direct ancestors. The first is of my great-great grandfather, Mariano Cruz: We do not know when he was born but he was from San Gabriel in the state of Andalusia in Spain. Among his ancestors were members of the Moorish population. In 1810, he came to Mexico. He was not a voluntary immigrant. In September of that year, the Mexican War of Independence began and lasted eleven bloody years. Mariano was a draftee in the Royal Spanish army and sent to Mexico to help put down the rebellion. Sometime between 1811 and 1818, he switched sides and joined the rebels, knowing that he would never be able to return to his family home in Spain and risking execution for desertion and treason if captured. In 1819, he married a native Mexican woman who was my great-great grandmother.

36

The other story is of my father, Antonio Cruz-Uribe: My father came to the United States in the year 1937. His primary motive was economics as he wanted to find a job that would enable him to get married and support a family. He settled in the city of San Antonio, Texas. While living there, he volunteered to help an individual who was running for mayor that had promised to make changes in the city government so that Mexicans would be treated "better."

One night there was a knock on his apartment door. When he opened the door, he saw a single man standing there. This individual spoke to my father in a calm and firm voice, saying: "Boy, you see that tree by the road?" pointing to a tree that stood in front of the apartment building. My father replied that he could see the tree. The man went on: "If you are still here tomorrow at this time, you will be swinging from that tree." The man turned away and left. That night, my father packed all his belongings into his car and fled from Texas.

In the previous years while he was living in Pachuca, Mexico, he had met a family from Antigo, Wisconsin who had come down to Mexico on vacation. Since he could speak English, he had acted as an interpreter for them. In return, they had told him on several occasions that if he was ever in the States to please stop by and visit. So, he drove to Wisconsin, a state that he barely knew the location of. After reaching the family, he told them what had happened. They helped him find a job in that area and he ended up moving to Green Bay, Wisconsin, when he got a better job at a company called Northwest Engineering where he was employed for 37 years.

As mentioned, my father worked for around 37 years for Northwest Engineering as an electrician (my father did attend some college in Mexico). In 1942, he was drafted by the U.S. army. He went to his boss (and this individual was my father's boss for another 30 years) and asked that he send a letter to the draft board requesting a deferment because my father was working in a defense required job (the company made cranes and other heavy equipment for the military). All his co-workers had such deferments. In fact, my father-in-law had such a deferment as a welder at Manitowoc shipyards during the same period. The draft board denied my father's application for a deferment. You have to draw your own conclusions, but it seemed quite obvious what was going on since my father was the only Mexican working at Northwest Engineering at that time and he was the only worker denied a deferment.

Since my father was a Mexican citizen, he refused to serve on grounds that he was not an American citizen. The draft board accepted that excuse but chose not to deport him. The only reason that I can guess was because he was working at a military necessary job. In fact, not long after this incident, the U.S. Army recruited him to join a group of people to study Japanese at St. Norbert's College and to work with radio intercepts. My father had started working with radios in the early 1920's and had a very desirable skill set in such electronics.

After the war, my father tried to become an American citizen but was denied because he had refused to serve in the military. During the xenophobia of the late 1940's and 1950's, the Immigration and Naturalization Services (INS) tagged my father as an undesirable and was going to deport him to Mexico even though he was married to an American woman and had five children who were all born in Green Bay, Wisconsin. The INS was stopped by Congressman John Byrnes, a Republican, in 1953. Yet, he warned my father that the INS may come back again.

Once again, in 1958, the INS came after my father. I do not know the exact reason for this, but it was very serious. Local friends of my parents who were associated with the new Wisconsin Senator, William Proxmire, had my father contact him. Even though Proxmire was new to the senate and only had met my father at this time, he went to the INS and (from my viewpoint) really twisted some arms. They agreed to drop all proceedings against my father and not to initiate any new ones in the future for any reason. However, it came with a price. My father was told that: One, he could never become an American citizen. Two, that he was allowed to live in the USA as a legal alien resident. Three, that he could only leave the country with the permission of the INS. And, four, that failing to get the proper permission, he would be denied entry back into the country or he would be deported if he was here.

Through connections with his friends in the Mexican government, my father was appointed the Counsel of Mexico to the State of Wisconsin in 1969. With that appointment came Diplomatic Immunity and this was recognized by then Secretary of State, William Rodgers. Now my father could travel freely without worry and the INS had no "control" over him. Among all his letters of congratulations for his appointment were those from the two U.S. Senators from Wisconsin, Gaylord Nelson and William Proxmire.

As the Counsel, my father always helped any citizen of Mexico that came to him who had "problems" with the INS (there were many). If they were working men with families, I know as a fact that my father went to great lengths to get them the documents they needed in order to get a green card or a legal residency. Years after my father passed away, I met on two separate occasions, individuals who owed their "wins" against the INS due to my father's interventions. One was the husband of my son's high school Spanish teacher. When I met her at a parent-teacher conference, she almost gave me a kiss and a hug in gratitude for what my father had done for her husband ten years before. At the time, I was not totally aware of these things as my father never talked about his dealings with the INS when he was Counsel. I understand why now. [9]

In Ben's telling of these stories, both the storyteller and audience become creatively involved in the re-imagining of events and moments of the protagonists' lives. Ben's stories contain universal and basic story elements that describe great personal challenges, responsible and caring actions, and a hope for reunion with loved ones that forecast happy endings for Mariano and Antonio, and their families. Further, as we hear or read stories like Ben's, we gain insight into the severe life-disruptions encountered, feel and re-experience the anxiety and cultural oppression endured, and feel inspired by the protagonists' courage and actions to protect and take care of others as they sought to live their lives with dignity and honor.

Eileen Johnson: A Story of Great Love and Resilience

In her storytelling, Eileen Johnson also describes the background of her family, conveying a strong familial bond with the actors that leads to insight and discovery of novel aspects of herself. Informed through Eileen's personal experiences and observations, as well as extensive genealogical research, here is her story:

> In 1763, John McDougall Johnston, Irish nobleman, left Ireland for America. He arrived in New York in 1790 and met an old friend in Montreal whose uncle was involved in the fur trade. The two left for Mackinac Island the following Spring. He was outfitted with all he would need for the winter and set out for the west. At last, they arrived at the Apostle Islands and, more specifically, Madeline Island. While wintering there, he met the daughter of the Ojibwe chief. After many months, and negotiating with her father, he was able to marry her and take her away from her tribal family. They eventually settled in the Soo (located in Sault Saint Marie, Michigan), building a home and starting a family which would one day include eight children. John continued to flourish in the fur trading business. His wife never learned English but did come to understand it. She was known as Neengay and The Woman of the Glade.
>
> The story of how John Johnston, native of Ireland, and Ozhah-guscodaywayquay, The Woman of the Glade, an Ojibwe chief's daughter, met and became man and wife

40

has more than enough romance and adventure for a story of the early days of the taming of this wild land. Indeed, their story is the story of the North Country and how it changed a native and a white man in the 19th and 20th centuries.

A portion of the homestead still stands almost 200 years later in the Soo. My cousins and I were able to visit this historic site within the past 3 years. There are still a few items from their time which are on display in this home. To walk over the yard, look over the rapids of the St. Mary's River site is breathtaking and inspiring. To imagine your ancestors once called this home. On the west side of the property, very near the house, there is a small overgrown garden which contains a statue of Neengay. She is shown as a young girl, kneeling in the glade. On her right shoulder sits an owl which indicates she is the daughter of a chief. Her left hand is cupped and holds blueberries. What a thrill it was to find that. Additionally, we were able to go inside a five-story Tower of History which overlooks the entire waterway which is Sault Saint Marie. At the uppermost story, there is a bronze plaque which memorializes these two people for their hospitality to all who came through that waterway and needed lodging and friendship.

What is to be learned from this great grandmother, about six-times removed? She was obedient to her father when he gave her to Johnston to be his wife. She was enduring. Leaving her family, heading to a new home many miles away, traveling long distances in an open canoe, becoming a wife to a foreigner whose language she did not speak. She also had to adjust to a permanent home, with a stove (not a fireplace which she was accustomed to), new foods, preparations to be made for the winter months, etc. Then along came the children, and her husband made months-long trips to the East, being gone for months on end. She managed the household during his absence and kept the family going. She was *resilient!*

Her youngest son, John McDougall Johnston, made his way southward as a fur trader and explorer, going as far as Gills Landing. This is where the story moves along and becomes closer to me. He took up with a Menominee woman, called Catishe, and thus we get closer to my grandmother, Mary Elizabeth Johnson, a generation or two later.

Mary Elizabeth Johnson was born in Keshena to an Indian woman and White man, Mary Ellen Weaver and Gustav Krueger. Her education included time at the local Indian Boarding School, Keshena Elementary, Tomah Indian Boarding School, and back to Shawano until she had finished eighth grade. In her late teens, she and a cousin made their way to Carlisle Indian School in Carlisle, Pennsylvania. This meant leaving her family and riding the train to eastern Pennsylvania. These boarding schools were established to "take the Indian out of the children." They came from all over the midwestern and western states, and Alaska. It was not unusual for them to be terrified of the big black train engine, belching smoke from its stacks and making terrifying sounds, that came to transport them to Pennsylvania. Many came simply wrapped in their Indian blankets and were taken by train to Carlisle. Imagine what a frightening experience this was for all of those little children, some as young as 6 or 7 years of age. A study of these schools is intense all by itself.

Grandma Johnson had gone with the intention of studying to become a teacher but had to leave the program early to care for her mother who was dying and her younger brother. Any career aspirations were ended.

As I've grown older, I can think that, in spite of the unpleasantness of Carlisle, she did learn some skills which served her for the rest of her life. As a wife and mother on a farm, she had to work hard, running the family, providing food, keeping a boarder, being involved in the Methodist Church, and other community activities. She was able to serve as president of the women's group at the church and in the American Legion Auxiliary. She could set a "nice" table; she canned and preserved the family's food; she could sew very well. The house had nice furniture and known prints of paintings hanging on the walls; one in particular we cousins remember is "Whistler's Mother." There was plenty of adversity that challenged her. She moved to Montana early in her marriage, they lost a child to drowning when he was only 2, two sons were missing in action at the same time during WWII. Her husband died at 66 and she was left to depend on her children for sustenance. She was *resilient!*

On my father's ancestral side, my Grandma Paulson came from Sweden to Chicago in the 1890's. She also left her family, changed her surname, came to a new land, didn't know the language, and had no education for a job. She worked for a short time at the World's Exposition in Chicago, met Albert Paulson (another Swede) and moved to northern Wisconsin. There they purchased land and farmed for a time. He later bought a tavern, where his son would eventually take over the business. She was also *resilient!*

No one walks through life without experiencing some very difficult challenges. My college consolidated with another, and I had to find my way at another campus. My husband died of cancer when he was 43. I was left with two small children at the age of 31. I had no job preparation. And so, I learned at an early age to draw strength to meet the demands of raising a family, keeping a home, making a social life, and making my way in a society where being a single parent is challenging. Eventually, I moved my little family to Green Bay, went back to school and graduated from the University of Wisconsin-Green Bay in 1984 with a music degree. I was 39. I was able to teach for the next 23 years, gaining a retirement fund. I remarried (to my grade school boyfriend) in 1997. He passed away in 2008, having had a double lung transplant. I can look back and say that I have had a rich life, filled with children, grandchildren, family, and friends. It is my hope that one day people will say of me—She was *resilient!*

I should note too, that as well as being resilient, there was the thread of education that sustained all these women and led to their successful survival in the midst of serious challenges. [10]

Like Ben's story we find universal and basic story elements that describe adversity and challenge, personal sacrifice, and the comfort of loving relationships. As we hear about the protagonists' lives, we become aware of the hardships they experienced, empathically respond to the unease they may have felt, and feel inspired by their gallant nature and steadfast quest to overcome. In Ben and Eileen's storytelling, they allude to their own personal growth, as new insights are grasped and integrated into their own life stories. They express an intergenerational exchange of the moral values of respect for the person and care for others beyond oneself, and celebrate a faith in the human family and a hope to overcome life's challenges. Certainly, these are characteristics that in their re-telling and hearing inspire us to continue to meet the many challenges of our current living.

As recognized in Ben and Eileen's stories, much like the chapters and sub-sections of each of our personal life stories, looking back on and reminiscing about our life provides us a way to affirm our self-worth, count blessings, and express a spirit of gratitude. Further, our self-reflection allows us to make adaptive adjustment as we seek to find ways to be happy as we continue in our life journey. Thus, how life-review, reminiscence and narrative processes are used therapeutically is discussed next.

A Closer Look at Life-Review, Reminiscence, and Narrative Therapy

As we mentioned in the last chapter, we often share with family and friends about the day's unfolding, reflecting on various past experiences and considering our next moments in life. These conversations, like the stories Ben and Eileen shared, reveal our deeper psychology in many ways, and our interest in "figuring out life." They also contain an assortment of "plots" and "key characters," and display our need to belong, to be recognized for our achievements, forgiven for our mistakes, and present to others the hopes and dreams we hold dearest. These opportunities for talking and sharing about our life often provide a tonic for the various calamities we experience, allowing us to gather the insight of others when we might need to rework, revise, or reestablish ourselves in our life journey. These benefits of sharing the story of our lives are also recognized in the therapeutic processes of life-review, reminiscence, and narrative therapy.

The American physician and gerontologist Robert Butler and social worker and psychotherapist Myrna Lewis first noted that older adults often are involved in looking back upon their life.[11] Thus, recognizing the importance of this self-reflection, the *life-review* was developed to facilitate a deeper understanding of self and gain a sense of integrity about the life one has lived. Moreover, it is suggested that the life-review process provides benefit in resolving past intrapersonal and interpersonal conflicts, and in enabling a transcendence forward in the last years, months, or weeks of life. However, this is a psychotherapy approach that may not be for everyone, as it seeks an uncovering and deep understanding of past life experiences, and special efforts are made to resolve issues surrounding feelings of guilt, bitterness, resentment, mistrust, dependency, and nihilism.[12] Various techniques to help dredge-up workable material and enter into the therapeutic life-review process may include analysis of written or orally recorded life-histories, or encouragement for the individual to take trips back to old neighborhoods and other places in the person's childhood or young adulthood, or to attend high school, college, family, or church reunions, to explore one's family tree and genealogical background, review of scrapbooks, photo albums, correspondences and other memorabilia. Other techniques include the development of a work history or an achievement resume, and activities that provide ways of preserving ethnic identity. The notion is that through these activities one may bring into discussion earlier dreams in life, find ways to accept personal failures, or ways of operating that may have made life difficult for the person or those around them. In doing so, life-review processes help facilitate an understanding of important values and ethics for living, and possible ways one may re-orient beliefs and change behaviors so that conflicts may be resolved. In addition, life-review processes may help the person discern and make provisions for the legacy that they wish to leave, as well as how to reckon with one's own mortality as death approaches. While the hoped-for outcome of this therapy is a greater integration of self and a resilience of spirit for living, there may also be moments of great emotional difficulty as one relives events and perhaps feels regret for choices made, or sadness because one senses their life has quickly passed and is now almost over. Thus, as noted previously, this is not an approach that would necessarily be used with individuals who lack requisite emotional resources to delve into difficult personal material or rework notions about one's purpose and life's meaning, or may in other ways be considered psychologically fragile.

Reminiscence refers to the recollecting of our life events and experiences. This person-centered therapy is often facilitated in a group setting. It is an approach that has wide-ranging application, and often not strictly bounded within theoretic or therapeutic formats.[13] It may include facilitating techniques such as singing songs or other types of musical therapy, using key words to elicit and trigger memories, as well as activities such as developing a life story book to help facilitate recollection of life events and experiences. Research suggests reminiscence therapy may enhance well-being, improve personal interactions, cognition, and lower anxiety and depressive symptoms.[14] It can be especially beneficial in helping individuals with dementia connect with their past, recall the mile-stone markers and major events of life, and experience a moment where they may express a sense of joy and vitality in their current living. Of all the "talk therapies," reminiscence is probably most like the casual discussions we have with family and friends where we may selectively share about our lives, and in some manner revise and continue to re-tell our story as we grow older.

Somewhat akin to life-review, *narrative therapy* is a discussion method that seeks to bring into focus a disruptive and enduring life-problem or difficulty, with the goal of establishing a dialogue that provides a new way to manage and overcome the problem or topic of concern.[15] This therapeutic approach is an alternative to traditional group psychotherapy, and involves three procedural phases: First, deconstructing the problem-story by seeing the problem or life-predicament objectively so that the problem is separate from the person. This deconstruction procedure allows for placing the problem or concern in another space in time, or colloquially, in a "past life," distinct from the person's living in the present moment. The second phase is authoring, where one revises their life story by adding new features that recognizes the problem as one aspect of a much more complex landscape. By becoming the author of their revised story, the person creates an alternate narrative with different plot-twists and a re-imagining of a different, more preferable outcome. The last phase of this therapeutic process is sharing. In this final procedure the person tells their revised story and discusses preferred outcomes and ways of living with others. As reported by researchers Paula Gardner and Jennifer Poole, narrative therapy has been successful in promoting resiliency in older individuals with depression and mental health problems, survivors of violence and trauma, and in providing support for deconstructing dominant sexist and cultural narratives.[16] These same researchers have also shown that life narrative therapy may be successful in working with individuals who grapple with the long-suffering problems of drug misuse and addiction. For example, as one older study participant who has battled addiction for many years reported, this method offers a new approach that through the deconstruction and revision of one's life story, and the therapeutic sharing with supportive others, can inspire the person to effectively deal with their problem and live more adaptively.[17]

Life Story Work

Incorporating many aspects of the approaches already discussed, *life story work* refers to the gathering of oral, written, or other information and artifacts that describe the person's life-history and cultural background, as well as current interests and concerns. In a selective review of the literature, life story work was noted to encompass a variety of facilitating methods, including appreciative personal inquiry, autobiographical interview, prompted group reminiscence, group improvisational and dramatic expression, sharing of one's life story in a group discussion, and personal journaling, as well as the composing of life-chapters, life story books, and web-pages.[18] This is also an approach that has found application across the age-spectrum, used with children, adolescents, young and older adults, and is suggested to help the individual gain a sense that they have been heard, and that their personal opinions and life matters.

With implications for wellness and disease management, life story work has been used world-wide as a component of interventions targeting cognition and memory, cancer, depression, heart disease, mental health, personal agency/autonomy, physical activity, physical pain, quality of life, resilience, and spiritual distress.[19] Importantly, telling one's life story to receptive listeners aids in the interpretation of the individual's quality of life, and in providing effective and appropriate care.[20] Moreover, the telling of one's life story increases communication between the person and caregiver; thereby allowing the caregiver to be more attuned to the person's concerns, their cultural background and practices, and, importantly, the person's individuality and uniqueness that are key in providing optimal care.[21] Yet, as we consider medical and other public and private settings, it should be noted that not all people may feel safe or comfortable discussing their background and sharing their life history.[22]

Life story work in the form of reminiscence and life-review has been found to aid the older adult as they seek to address existential concerns and find adaptive resolution.[23] One topic of particular importance is loss. A loved one's illness and death are important events that can bring about a compassionate re-evaluation and understanding of one's life and the losses endured.[24] Through this type of reminiscing, it is hoped a re-balancing and acceptance may take place. This reinterpretation of life events and finding new meaning reflects a growth orientation that is frequently recognized both as an essential process, and as a significant consequence of life story work.[25] Beyond the facilitation of reminiscence, life-review, and re-interpretive processes, other associated benefits of various forms of life story work used in wellness and disease management include the reduction of depressive symptoms, pain intensity, heightened well-being, and increased opportunity for physical activity.[26]

Creatively, the production of a legacy object (e.g., a photo album, scrap book, memory box, or memory book) as a method to share one's life story is recognized to facilitate communication of the elder's unique history with family and caregivers, and in its construction offers another avenue for discovering personal meaning and purpose in life.[27] The use of life story books and group sharing are especially effective in promoting a sense of personhood and improving communication and social relationships for individuals with dementia and intellectual disability.[28] Thus, in its broad approach and therapeutic application, life story work provides a way for the person to talk about their life, and a way for family members and friends to know about and celebrate the person and the life they have lived. We will continue to consider how we may find self-discovery in creative activities in later chapters, but let's now consider how we might also tell our story and celebrate our living via another method of creative expression, weaving and fiber works.

Self-Discovery and Celebration of the Many Threads of Our Creativity

Like our life story, our creative expressions convey a rich narrative about who we are and where we came from, and reflect our hopes and dreams for what might yet be and what is still possible. As we begin to look closer at other forms of creative expressions, perhaps one of the most incomparable examples to consider is that of American fiber artist Consuelo Jimenez Underwood.

Born in Sacramento, California, the eleventh of twelve children to a Chicana mother and Huichol Indian father, early in her life Consuelo Jimenez Underwood and her family worked as migrant farmers throughout California. To avoid deportation of her father who was a citizen of Mexico, the family maintained homes both in Mexicali, Mexico, and in the cross-border town of

Calexico, California. As an aspiring young artist, Consuelo was influenced by her father's interest in weaving, and the woven dresses he made for her to wear as a little girl. A talented student, Consuelo received her B.A. and M.A. from San Diego State University, and artistically inspired, she received her M.F.A. and later joined the faculty and headed the Fiber Area at San Jose State University until her retirement in 2009. Throughout her career, Consuelo's creative work and teaching helped to establish and gain recognition for weaving and fiber works as a bona fide art form. Considering again how one's personal history informs their later development, Consuelo's life and art allows us insight into the plight of immigrant peoples, the meaning of "crossing over the border," and how fiber arts may symbolically reflect important life-themes and developmental concerns. Now in her 70s, describing self-discoveries and celebrations in later life, here is Consuelo's story:

> In the seventh decade of my life, I have a whole new way of looking at the world. It is like I am rediscovering myself. At the age of nine I was inspired by Joan of Arc and how she stood up to the trials she faced, as at the age of fourteen she led an army to kick England out of France. I cried when I read her story because I had a similar challenge. In terms of self-awareness, I recognized the cultural and social barriers that excluded families like mine. I could see there was another world on the other side of those barriers. My challenges were how do I understand this other world, and how do I ride pass those barriers and infiltrate that world? I found out as a young person that it was through education. Yet, it was like going to war. I learned that in physical sports that I could pretty much be a star. When playing board games, I would inevitably lose. In Chess I found out I could beat anybody. So, I told myself, don't rely on luck to help you, use your Chess expertise! I did not make the social barriers a part of myself. In my self-awareness I wanted to overcome and get past thinking about having this or that status in life. I knew that whatever I needed to do, I could

do—that if I needed my eyes to look further, they could—If I needed my legs to run faster, they could. The cultural and social barriers were just like a plank that I could jump off of—that I could jump high above the plank and over the water below.

In my life now, what excites me are all the challenges that I have yet to overcome. It is like seeing a mountain, and then you climb it. Then you see another mountain, and you climb that one. And now I have the understanding that the approach to the mountains is different at ages nine, and twenty, and forty, and sixty. And all of a sudden, now at age seventy, just saying "because there is a mountain there and that I will climb it"—I don't think so. There is no time— I am very aware of my path, and that from my place in my family ... I knew that I was so far down that I could only go up. So that inspired me. What now do I want to prove? Well, I want everyone to know about the horrific border that we had to cross as a family and had to go back and forth over to live. I hated that border so much that I knew that when I grew up I was going to do something. So, in college I studied art and got a degree—but I entered academia with a needle and thread, and with the intention of taking the border between art and craft down! Congruently, I was going to inform the viewer about border issues.

My Dad weaved when there was no work because of the rain. He had a loom in the garage. He would weave simple dresses for me to wear. But by the time I was seven he stopped weaving because other family members would come and see him weaving and ridicule him, saying "weaving is for women" and that got me so angry. I thought, how dare they laugh at him because he is weaving. Later in Art History class they were showing all these beautiful, woven fabrics, and I thought my Dad did this! I am going to pick up the thread and needle and I am going to make art with it!

In 1981 I was the only graduate student in fiber... and I knew that all the things I had been challenged by could become my strengths... and thus my work is seen as radical... but I have to make two or three pieces a year...because my art is from the Gods and I have a lot of ideas in my mind and I think that if I don't make those pieces then I am letting Them and the ideas down and I feel bad—so I always have two or three projects going.

But as an artist I can do anything I want—I have absolute freedom—so let's tear that wall down that labels different creative expressions as an "art" or a "craft.' That is easier than tearing down the border between Mexico and the U.S. So, my work was easy. All I had to do was manipulate that thread to make people say "huh?" To think and go "wow!"[29]

Indeed, Consuelo's weaving is provocative in its portrayal of both very beautiful as well as horrific aspects of life that many people might prefer to look away from, or simply ignore. Further, her art summons forth an interpretation that requires inner reflection and deeper inquiry into social biases, ethnic and racial discrimination, social justice, and ways we might embrace equality for all persons. A particularly well recognized work is a quilt that is held at the Smithsonian Museum entitled, *Virgen de los Caminos*. This art piece draws attention to the many dangers that people from other countries encounter when they come to find work in the United States. In the center of its white background is the embroidered robed skeletal figure of the Virgen, an intercessor and symbolic figure much like that of the Virgin of Guadalupe, patron Goddess of Mexico. Swathed across the quilt and the Virgen de los Caminos are strands of barbed wire, an especially poignant "thread" that reflects communal separation, threats to individual freedom, and the personal injury of borders. Around the edges of the quilt are embroidered beautiful flowers of many colors—symbols of innocence, anticipation, overcoming, pride, and hope. Throughout the background, a veiling white thread portrays the recurring image of a man with a mustache, a woman wearing a dress, and

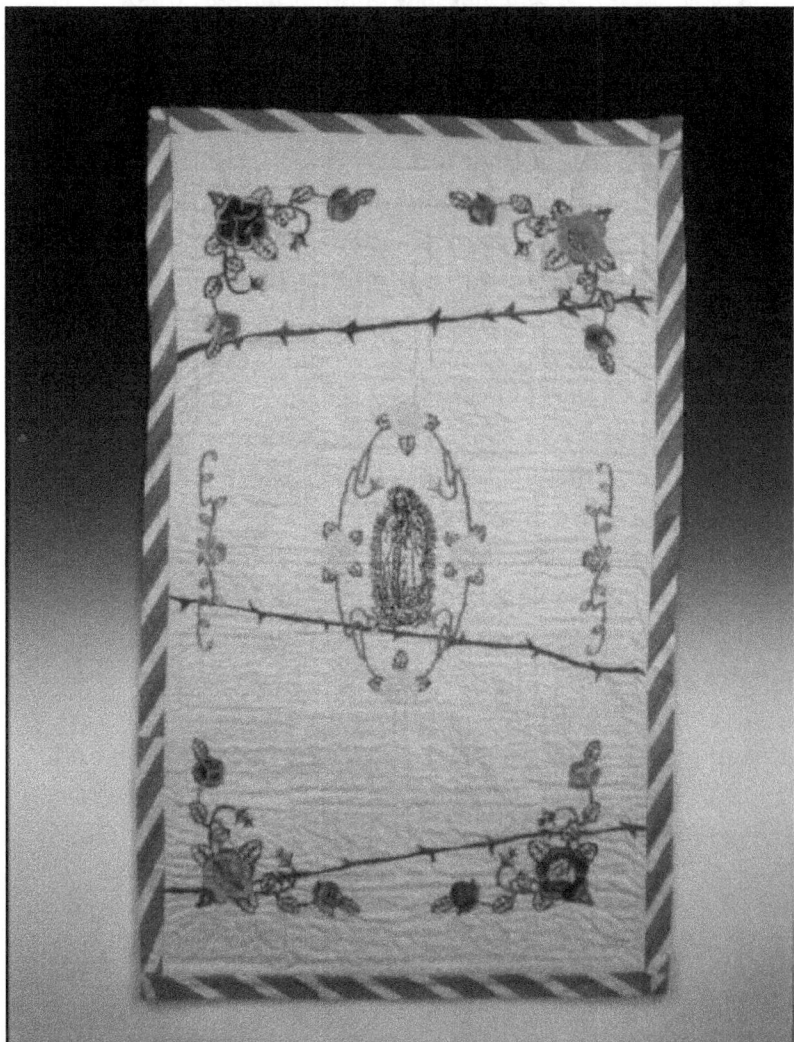

Figure 3.1: *Consuelo Jimenez Underwood, Virgen de los Caminos, 1994, embroidered and quilted cotton and silk with graphite, Smithsonian American Art Museum, Museum purchase, 1996.77. Digital image courtesy of Smithsonian American Art Museum.*

their young daughter with her hair in pigtails, all desperately running and holding hands as they cross the road. This motif is similar to the road-signage developed and used by the California

Department of Transportation, warning of immigrants crossing from the border, and a key element in other works by the artist.

In another of her works entitled, *Run, Jane, Run!* Consuelo expresses the xenophobia and anti-immigrant attitudes prevalent in American culture.[30] Intended to highlight the stereotypical caricature of Mexican immigrants, this work explicitly depicts a road sign found in the Southwest United States, that has been recognized to espouse the dehumanization of migrants by depicting them similar to animals, and a characterization of the Mexico-U.S. border that members of the California legislature used to create legislation in California that would bar immigrants from receiving public health services or from entering the public education system.[31] Truly, these exquisite and profound works by Consuelo Jiménez Underwood reflect the masterful techniques of a great American artist.[32] But what is more, works such as *Virgen de los Caminos* and other weavings by Consuelo call our attention to the absurdity of violence that emanates from prejudice, discrimination, and exclusion, and the need for mutual respect and equality for all people.

In her early seventies, Consuelo Jiménez Underwood is recognized world-wide, and she remains active as an artist and teacher, developing new pieces for exhibit and offering teaching workshops for students. On everyday life Consuelo remarks:

> I can't wait to get up in the mornings to continue my work... but I still have to deal with the mundane aspects of life... like paying bills and taxes! I retired after 20 years of teaching... but I am still very much involved in my work— I am still playing Chess and hoping to say "Checkmate!" with my work... I still have seven more years I hope to do my work, and then I will evaluate what is next...

Reflecting on the purpose of her art, Consuelo noted:

> All I want to do is inform... everyone has these issues... all nations have these issues, and so my job is to inform—the struggle is real. The world is beautiful—and we are caught

in the middle—what are we going to do? What are you going to do?

Expressing a cosmic consciousness, and suggesting a deeper meaning and purpose to be discovered in later life, Consuelo offers us insight into the allegory of her artwork:

> I make art for the wind, for the clouds. I just made one for the birds, and now I feel better—they are happy now…
> There is always hope, there is always struggle… we are in the middle of it… It is different for each person, but in the Toltec culture the philosophy is that we should make flowers and songs… I will continue my dreaming and journey and share my insights with the world.

In her art, where each thread has an essential importance and meaningfulness, Consuelo reminds us that each person has equal significance and purpose in the tapestry of life.

Celebrating Our Story

In our storytelling we tell others about ourselves, our families, and the experiences that have made us into the people we have become. When we share the inspirational stories of family members, friends, and others, we announce other ways of seeing and being in the world. We express and convey our dreams for the future. As recognized in the stories of Ben, Eileen, and Consuelo, we also express a celebration of life. Indeed, in sharing our stories we travel upon a creative avenue that leads us to find new hope, meaning, and purpose in our living, and to celebrate the story of our life.

FOUR — TRANSITIONS AND EXISTENTIAL CONCERNS THROUGHOUT THE LIFE-COURSE

In fourth grade, at the end of the school year, one of the author's school band director informed the band that on the last day of school they would assemble on the playground outside the elementary school and perform a marching concert. Band members were instructed to wear white shirts and slacks, and their band uniform's red cape and hat. Not only was this the last day of school, but it was also a special day. It was the band's "first" concert and performance of all the pieces they had been practicing over the spring. As the band gathered on the playground there was an electricity about the moment. Their uniforms expressed majesty and celebration. The students were proud to be dressed so nattily, and excited about the performance that would soon occur. The band formed in marching ranks, and while standing stationary, at the conductor's direction began the first piece, an exciting march by John Phillip Sousa. Performing outdoors, the music articulated the great fanfare of the beginning of summer. The melody was jubilant and voiced the students' collective joy of performing. Throughout all the rehearsals, the band had never sounded this good! It seemed like the sounds of flutes, clarinets, brass instruments, and percussion shared the countenance of the sun's warmth and illuminating glow, and the sweet harmony of the gentle breeze we felt that day! There was also the strong sense that this was a defining moment—the realization that the young student was also a "musician." This understanding would become a facet of how the fledgling musician would construct a sense of self and form an identity in the ensuing years. Thus, to paraphrase the old saying, "you can take the person out of the band, but you can't take the band out of the person." When we think about the concepts of self and identity, we recognize the diversity that they may represent for each of us personally. We are made up of a lot of things. For example, our sense of self, and in many ways our deeper psychological identity, is a product of how we are known by others. Moreover, as the famous psychologist William James earlier suggested, we have as many facets of self as there are people who hold an image of us in their minds.[1] Embracing the whole person approach, we realize too that we are more than the sum of all the parts that make up concepts of self and identity. From this orientation we understand our "selves" and others in a way that recognizes enduring traits, familial origins and environmental influences that combine to direct our thinking and acting. But there is also an awareness of the many possibilities that exist for each of us as well, and what we might yet become in our living. So, while early experiences like playing in a band are moments that may instill an initial sense of pride and identity, and foster and contribute to a conscious way of knowing oneself, they also illuminate the infinite dimensions of each of us. Thus, in whatever creative activity you pursue and by whatever painter's smock or orchestra attire you wear, as William James suggests, you are recognized and known by these activities; that is, as a painter, sculptor, singer, musician, needle-pointer, or artist or craftsperson of other sorts.

Life Transitions: Existential Concerns in Childhood

As Erik Erikson notes in his theory of psychosocial development, early in life our first concerns involve resolving the crises of trust versus mistrust, and developing a sense of personal autonomy and initiative.[2] Positive and healthy parent-child interactions within the first years of life promote a sense of hope, as well as the freedom and encouragement to explore and make an impact upon the world. Moreover, caregivers provide key support and models of creative expression, social communication, and regulation of emotions that aid us in our earliest development. Our physical, cognitive, and socioemotional growth continues throughout early childhood, as do existential concerns.[3] Thus, moms and dads and other important members of the social network (e.g., teachers, grandparents, siblings, friends) play critical roles in helping children to frame and address existential questions such as "Can I trust the world?," "Is it okay to be me?," and, "Is it okay for me to do, move, and act?"[4] Thus, the stories children tell in early childhood express their unique egocentric perspective and relate

57

what they feel (e.g., what is comforting, what is scary), what they think (e.g., recollection of events, what they like), what they can do (e.g., dance, sing, sleep, play), and how they understand the world (e.g., who is in charge, what is fair).[5] Certainly, the way parents interact with and raise children is associated with the child's social competency and self-control, as well as success in dealing with the existential concerns that arise.[6]

Problems and difficulties encountered in childhood may affect development and learning later on. This is an important concern for parents and teachers as they hope to assist each child in reaching their greatest potential. The time of middle childhood often involves gaining a sense of and feeling more grown-up. For some children, the tenth birthday becomes the "Big-One-O" and represents a milestone and crossing-point into the preteen years and greater responsibility. As we look globally, for some children the end of the first decade of life might mean a time to leave school to work, or to carry-out assigned roles within the family.[7] For many children, there may be real and thus stark awareness of poverty, food and housing insecurities, racism, ethnic oppressions, and warfare that they endure, and the existential threat that any of these represent. The trauma of these events and other adverse childhood experiences (the incarceration, mental illness, or death of a parent, being a victim of sexual assault, or witnessing domestic violence, etc.), are likely to be so distressing that they present anxieties that may last a lifetime.[8]

Important concerns in later childhood and at the dawn of adolescence include a more differentiated understanding of self (e.g., developing a positive self-concept and self-esteem), emotions, life-stressors, and the influence of friends and peers. This is also a time of industry versus inferiority in Erikson's psychosocial development theory, representing another early existential concern for the developing person. How the child sees themselves in relation to peers, assists the child in gaining a sense of esteem about their skills and current capabilities. Further, academic struggles or failures convey a social status early on about the individual that is influenced and affected by peer-relationships. Lagging behind peers in physical or intellectual development can have detrimental effects on the child's self-esteem. Indeed, researchers suggest that children who lag behind peers in academic areas, especially in reading, are likely to develop very negative views of self and thus have poor self-esteem.[9] Literacy (i.e., the ability to read and write) is a doorway to many avenues in life, and research has suggested that poor-reading skills and illiteracy predict many problems in adolescence and adulthood.[10] Reflecting the great imagination of children and the dreams about life that have directed their play, key existential questions of later childhood include, "How do I compare with other kids?," "What am I good at?," and, "Can I make it in the world of people and things?"[11] Resultantly, in later childhood children tell more elaborate stories that convey information about their special talents and struggles, express unidirectional and reciprocal patterns of social exchange, depict cultural and gender-oriented parameters of their socialization, as well as their dreams and fantasies of what adulthood and later times in development will be like for them.[12]

Life Transitions: Existential Concerns in Adolescence and Young Adulthood

Puberty sets in motion dramatic physical, cognitive, and socioemotional changes that begin a transition into adulthood. This can also be a time that is rather volatile and risky for the individual. With physical changes come the recognition of a new body image, different from that of childhood, and exploration of sexuality. In general, adolescence might be regarded as a time of many firsts, such as a first date, a first job, and a time where there is easier access to alcohol, tobacco, and other substances, as well as increased risk for sexual misadventures, illegal activities, school failure, and mental health problems. Moreover, these latter challenges and negative experiences may besiege the person and promote an "existential dread" about life itself.[13]

Adolescence is also a time of novel perspective taking and thinking that is similar to the hypothetical deductive reasoning of scientists. It is also a time where there is new emphasis and concern about oneself in relation to others. As Erik Erikson describes, the central crisis of this stage of development involves forming an identity versus role confusion. Similarly, existential concerns include addressing questions of "Who am I?" and, "Who can I be?"[14] The personal story told is also more complex, often expressing the expectations and divergent pressures to conform from family, peers, and society, as well as the complexity of establishing one's identity.[15] To grow into young adulthood means to become autonomous, but to still be connected to one's family and community. This is easier said than done for many, as we recognize that adolescence is often a time where parent-child discord is at its peak. When you stop and think about it, we can all probably recall a time when we were in conflict with parents or knew someone who was. Thus, during our teen years we begin to grow beyond our families, confiding more in friends than parents. Further, with expanding patterns of socialization come opportunities for new social roles and the formation of intimate relationships.

As we transition into young adulthood, one notion we might entertain is that we are ready for life's "prime time." Yet, we are likely to have not completely resolved important life-questions like what work will I do for a living or when will I form a family? Thus, as we begin to live independently and find a place in the adult world, we realize there is no "User's Manual" available to assist us. We will just have to work through life's challenges as we encounter them. As a result, young adulthood is a very stressful time, and accordingly we see high rates of mental illness such as depression, general anxiety disorder, alcohol and other substances abuse, and schizophrenia.

Signaling changes that become more common place as we get older, in young adulthood there is often a decline from the peak levels of physical fitness in our middle and late teen years. Indeed, the body's metabolism is slowing, and while most of us are no longer growing taller there is a tendency to expand through the mid-section, with a few pounds added each year as we progress into middle age. The greatest health risks during young adulthood come in the form of physical inactivity, substance abuse, and sexually transmitted infection. Many young adults express an optimistic bias about their likelihood of encountering these problems—that "it won't happen to me!" thinking—even though the same individuals may be involved in behaviors such as binge drinking, drug use, or tobacco use, all of which increase the risk for health problems in the future. But wishful thinking is just that, wishful thinking. The scientific data reveal the real scope of the problem, and makes clear that young adults should be very concerned about risk for obesity (e.g., over 30% of U.S. adults fall in the obese category), binge-drinking and the slippery-slope that leads to alcoholism (e.g., 40% to 50% of men in the U.S. engage in binge drinking throughout their twenties) and acquiring sexually transmitted infections (e.g., about 3 million people in the U.S. are infected with Chlamydia annually).[16]

In young adulthood we acquire many new powers of mind. Indeed, we can think and process information faster, and may shift during early adulthood from an absolutist way of thinking (e.g., right or wrong) to a more relativistic orientation that considers multiple perspectives.[17] This is also a time of greater creativity and creative expression. Furthermore, in young adulthood there is the beginning of commitments to careers and full-time jobs to pay one's own way, caring for a family, and contributing to the broader community. Erikson proposes the psychosocial crisis at this stage of development is intimacy versus isolation. Indeed, addressing the existential question "Can I love?", and forming and maintaining of an intimate connection are concerns that shape our personal story throughout adulthood.[18] Marriages and partnerships have unique challenges and great benefits. Some of the challenges that seem to be "deal breakers" are lack of communication, drug use by one or both partners, and infidelity. Perhaps the most significant new experience in young adulthood is becoming a spouse, or a parent. These events change one's orientation very dramatically (e.g., there is a new role: you're a husband, wife, or partner; you are called Mom or Dad, and there are new responsibilities too!).

Nonetheless, the awareness that many dreams about what life would bring or would be like may never be realizable, and the struggle to make a life for oneself as avenues of opportunity begin to narrow and close-off, bring into awareness the existential questions, "How can I make a 'real' living and have a good paying job? Who can I share my life with? How will I take care of my family? What is possible for us now? What will life bring? What kind of 'future' can we construct?" These critical questions may be more pragmatic but evolve from how earlier challenges have been met and resolved that allows the person to hold hope for the future. These concerns also anchor and add to the richness of our personal narrative as we describe our life's story and continue into middle and later adulthood.[19]

Life Transitions: Existential Concerns during Middle and Later Adulthood

Development continues into middle and later adulthood. Thus, at midlife we note changes in hair (e.g., first signs of graying, and thinner hair if not baldness), skin (e.g., wrinkles), and joints (e.g., loss of thickness of cartilage for most of us, first stages of arthritis for many). If you've been involved in an exercise routine, you may have maintained or slowed your loss of muscle mass and strength somewhat. You will have likely lowered your risk for age-related diseases such as cardiovascular disease and diabetes. At midlife, we also note an increase in diagnosis of early signs of chronic disorders, and, perhaps in retrospect, become profoundly aware that poor lifestyle choices earlier in adulthood (e.g., smoking, lack of exercise, use of intoxicants) have powerful influences on health later in life. With advancing age, there is an increased risk for a variety of diseases. Indeed, the leading causes of death at midlife and older age are cancer, heart disease, cerebrovascular and pulmonary diseases. For women, menopause occurs. For men too, a decline in testosterone production occurs that may mimic the loss of estrogen production in women and can affect sexual activity. However, just as intimacy and romance has been a part of one's life in young adulthood, physical contact and sexual expression are still important interests at midlife as well. All these physical changes and concerns for health and well-being bring new existential concerns to light and pose many new questions about how we might survive and what is yet possible in life.

At midlife, we also experience subtle changes in sensory-perceptual systems (e.g., decline in hearing sensitivity, visual acuity) due to the natural declines and wear-and-tear on the biological mechanisms that underlie these systems. Of note is a decline in fluid intelligence (i.e., an aspect of intellectual capability that reflects the neurological integrity of brain systems), but maintenance and perhaps even slight increase in crystallized intelligence (i.e., an aspect of intellectual capability that reflects educational background and experience) as we age. In general, our ability to think and process information is gradually slowing, and working with novel problems becomes more challenging at midlife. Yet, this is a time when we may be our most creative, and at the peak of our career and work life.

Midlife is also a time when we become more aware of our own finite existence. Psychiatrist Carl Jung and personality theorist Bernice Neugarten both have suggested midlife as a time of turning inward, where we seek a deeper understanding of life's meaning and purpose.[20] Spirituality and religious activities can provide an answer to these questions. Thus, there seems to be an increased interest in and expression of spirituality as one transcends from early adulthood to midlife and then into later adulthood. Erik Erikson proposes generativity versus stagnation as the central psychosocial crisis of midlife. Generativity refers to the caregiving and concern we provide and express to children, older family members and friends, as well as institutions and organizations in our communities. Stagnation reflects a regression to an earlier status of isolation and lack of social connection. Accompanying existential concerns are voiced in questions such as, "Can I make a difference?" and, "Does my life matter?"[21] The personal story at midlife then often includes more elaborated concerns about health, well-being, communal relationships and prosocial actions, filtered through generative and self-actualizing or stagnant and regressive ego stances.[22]

As previously noted, in later life, risk for disease and declines in health become a greater part of our everyday experience and concern. We see increased prevalence of dementia, depression, and other diseases in older age. Prevention and early treatment may offer the best hope for the individual and family members in holding off the occurrence of these age-associated pathologies. Certainly, however, how we age reflects genetic inheritance (e.g., if grandparents and parents were long lived, we will likely be too) as well as lifestyle factors that influence health (e.g., smoking, diet rich in fats, and high stress jobs are associated with earlier mortality). Exercise, proper diet, and enriched environments help to slow declines in cognitive and physical capabilities, but do not stop this progression. In general, while there are changes and declines in sensory-perceptual processes and cognitive function with advancing age, there is also considerable individual variability. When various declines occur, how do we maintain a vital involvement in life? The answer seems to turn on our psychological approach to living and how we view our own development. Staying engaged in creative activities and pastimes, maintaining social connections, and having a positive outlook on life is likely to aid us in keeping to our exercise routines, following healthy nutritional guidelines, and staying intellectually active and vitally involved.

As you look through the family photo albums and see parents and grandparents when they were younger, you might recognize that they were a lot like you at an earlier age. Indeed, as we continue to mature, in many ways we begin to have more in common with older adults than we do with children and adolescents. What we expect from our relationships with others may change as well. Perhaps over time, we sense a personal shifting from "I can do it all by myself," to "I can use a little help with this," or vice versa. Or having the sense that one does not need to control all the details of life, even if one ever could. There are also new roles to enjoy, such as being a grandparent, and others that we might shun, like being a resident in a convalescent center or nursing home, that influence self-concept and what we might consider as possible ways of being.

Therefore, a central existential concern is our own aging. How we will live in later life, along with the notion of how to stay socially connected and involved in our work, and whether we are "using it or losing it" are important questions to address. In older age, life often becomes simpler in some ways (e.g., retirement from the hassles of work, time to do activities that you enjoy, more time to spend with family), but also more complex in others (e.g., worrying about or managing illness, confronting declines in intellectual abilities, caregiving for a spouse or partner). At this time in life, Erik Erikson suggests the central psychosocial crisis in older age is integrity versus despair. As a complement to Erikson's model, Tornstam has added an extension called gerotranscendence, where we prepare for the end of life.[23] Both of these aspects of later life address a form of the question we first posed earlier in adolescence: What identity will I choose so that life has meaning and purpose? But now in retrospect we ask: How has my life been purposeful and meaningful? Can I look back upon my life with a sense of integrity? Are the earlier standards of achievement still appropriate for me? As I consider my life in a transcendent way, what is my connection with processes of living and dying? Thus, in older age our personal story may tell of changes in one's self-concept and life-goals, and the deeper insights and understandings we have attained.[24] However, our personal story is likely to be silhouetted against a background of ageism and age discrimination that foster additional existential concerns for us in later life.

Thus, perhaps the most difficult "course" we ever enroll in is called, "learning about life," which culminates with its most challenging topic, "death." All throughout life we have become very familiar with death and grieving, as we have seen family members and friends die. Death is the ultimate existential concern, and a topic that we will come to know more and more about as we continue in our life journey.[25] As we grow closer to the time of our own death, we will seek to find ways to adapt and make sense of our lives and the world in which we live. Our critical questions may be more contemplative, but again evolve from and influenced by how we worked through earlier existential life-challenges. At the end of life we may communicate hope, compassion, and love as we creatively express ourselves and become immersed in transcendent concerns that connect us with all of nature and the flow of life.

Creative Response to Life's Existential Challenges

Throughout life we act creatively when we communicate our personal story. In our early life, however, how we grew as a person was supported by caring parents and others who imagined along with us what might be possible.[26] But as we grow into midlife and older age, our own imagination plays a much more central role in directing how we may pursue "possible dreams for our life," and how we will meet the existential challenges we encounter.[27] In the following interview with Victoria Jicha, she tells of her early life, and how in adulthood she met life challenges by discovering a variety of creative pathways that involved music, teaching, editorial writing, starting a music publication business, and becoming a Master Hand Knitter.

Victoria Jicha's Story

I grew up in a small-town west of Portland, Oregon. My mother was a musician and pianist, and my father a biology teacher. When I began playing the piano pieces I was hearing my mother's piano students play, she started me on piano lessons, I was 3. By the fifth-grade, band program instrument selection time, she had accepted my hands were too small to be the hands of a professional pianist. So, it was time to choose a different instrument. My mother had always loved the big flute solo in Brahms 1st symphony, so that was the instrument I started to play.

Just before high school there was a nationwide competition for scholarships to study at the National Woodwind Workshop at Lake Tahoe, NV. I prepared a tape, submitted it, and won the opportunity to study with Julius Baker, then principal flute of the New York Philharmonic Orchestra. This was my first exposure to a professional flutist of international stature. I flew into Reno – my first plane trip. I'll never forget it. Young ladies still wore hats and gloves and their Sunday-best when travelling in those days. My mother arranged for the local Episcopal priest to meet my plane and drive me up to Lake Tahoe. That boggles my mind when I think about it now.

The following fall I auditioned for the oldest youth orchestra in the US, the Portland Junior Symphony (now called the Portland Youth Philharmonic). I was in the 7th grade. That orchestra played a complete, standard, traditional orchestra repertoire. Some of the works I performed included Carl Orff's Carmina Burana, Brahms 2nd Symphony, and Tchaikovsky's 4th symphony. In my final year with them I performed the Ibert Concerto for flute and won a full scholarship to attend the Aspen Music Festival in Aspen Colorado. There I studied with Albert Tipton, who was principal flute in the Detroit Symphony. The following year I entered Oberlin College, and then married and transferred to Indiana University, where I graduated with a Bachelor of Music degree.

After two years living in Minneapolis, where my husband was the assistant principal flutist, we moved to Chicago where I got the job as 2nd flute in Grant Park Orchestra. While in Chicago (30+ years) I played with several Chicago orchestras, played in pit orchestras for musicals, and concentrated on chamber music, in and around the Chicago area. I also earned a Master of Church Music degree on organ at Northwestern University and held several positions with churches and synagogues. That led to a temporary position teaching harpsichord at Northwestern University, some solo work around town on harpsichord, and eventually the flute position teaching at Wheaton College.

I also taught flute in a full-time position at DePaul University, eventually becoming Chair of the Performance Department. I only mention this because it was unusual for a woman to hold such a position at that time. While I was teaching at DePaul, the school offered a computer buy-in program via payroll deduction for all faculty. I signed up and soon created a music publishing company. I founded Music Makers, Inc., and began transcribing orchestral works for flute choir. By the time I sold the company there were over 40 items in the catalogue and I had won several flute choir publishing awards. What I was doing required the ability to look at music on the page and hear it in your head without it being audible to others. I've always been able to do that.

The free-lance work in Chicago and relationships I developed while volunteering with the newly established National Flute Association introduced me to many people and that led to my final career position, Editor of *Flute Talk* magazine. I'm convinced I was hired for that job because of who I knew; I had no training as a writer other than good high school English teachers. That job opportunity came along just when I was discovering that my performing abilities were changing. The arthritis was beginning to take hold and the writing was on the wall. I played my last recital at Wheaton, walking off the stage unable to feel my hands.

This was my first big transitional accommodation. I was playing less flute, but was writing about it and working with flute players from around the world. Simultaneously I still had a church job where I was working with a volunteer choir and practicing organ every day. Working with a volunteer choir is a unique challenge that I always enjoyed a lot. Producing beautiful music out of 20-30 untrained singers who just love to sing is a high goal and depends a great deal on choosing the right anthems for their abilities. That's half the battle. Anyway, I was pretty good at it and had a lot of fun.

The second transition and accommodation occurred when my husband was transferred to Humana's Green Bay office. It came at a good time, as my career was winding down anyway. I worked for the magazine from Green Bay for a couple of years and eventually retired in 2014.

Shortly after we moved to Green Bay a Joann Fabrics store opened up. I remember standing in the checkout line and seeing a knitting magazine. I picked it up and discovered it was the house magazine of The Knitting Guild Association and they had a certification program advertised in the magazine to be a Master of Hand Knitting. I thought that might be a new direction to approach; I could teach in a local yarn store. So, I enrolled; it was a 3-year program, and I worked through the requirements. When I finished the program, I was the only Master Hand Knitter in Wisconsin. There are three others now.

I joined the local knitting guild and later discovered an active embroidery group locally here in Green Bay and in Appleton, Wisconsin. Retirement for me has been a series of downgrades, small changes, accommodations. I now have a list of UFOs (unfinished objects) needlecraft projects waiting for my attention. [28]

Suggesting the existential challenge that occurs when you have thought of yourself as a flutist and musician for 70 years or more, and you sense you are losing that identity, Victoria noted thinking, "If I am not a flutist, what am I?" Her story reflects a profound example of the guiding support of parents and teachers, how our interests may shift as we grow and mature, and how we may take a new tack later in life that allows for continued expression and fulfillment of creative interests. As Victoria notes, the transitions and accommodations we make across the life-course also involve imagining ourselves in new ways as we seek resolution to the existential questions we encounter.[29]

Back to the Garden

As we transcend through later adulthood, we may come upon existential questions concerning what we might still do and the ultimate purpose of our life.[30] Looking to resolve these questions we may turn to painting, sculpture, prose writing, playing music, or starting a new business, and in these creative activities find the source of our being. It is part of us. We share it with others. It abides with us. Through our creative actions, and at each stage in life, we push further into the discovery of ourselves. As contemplated and described by Herman Hesse's character Sinclair in his coming-of-age novel *Demian*, our perceptions, dreams, and interpretations of life-experiences have always mirrored back to us who we are.[31] Our discovery of this awareness and of our deeper psychology leads us back to the source. To the garden—a place of happiness, joy, comfort, and of love, hope, and respite, where we can encounter and imagine what is yet possible for us. It is a place that allows us to be who we are meant to be. But how do we start? How do we get back to the garden? It may mean listening to a new or different type of music, walking to the beat of your own drumming, picking up a musical instrument again or learning a new one, or taking a class in painting or ceramics. It might involve joining a community theatre group or blogging poetry or opinion articles on social media. Remarkably, most of us can make music, draw, and dance. We also travel on the great avenues of our creativity when we talk—it's in the glides and glissandos we use to accent and emphasize important words when we speak; in the syncopated expressions we use to convey special meaning in our conversations; in the beginning and ending of our phrases and the pauses we take to breath and relax; and, in the punctuations of our communications with a smile or look of surprise. It is in our walk too—as we move across the room; in the striding cadence of our exercise march; in the careful and choreographed steps we take when we meet and greet friends. So being creative is easy. Keep the pulse or play off the beat as you accompany a song or the orchestra. Paint abstractly or draw caricatures that portray the joyful as well as the darker aspects of life. Write from your heart and share your cultural perspective. Begin a new job or start your own business. But be gentle with yourself. Drink in the reverberations of this new music. Explore your deepest feelings as you write your new poem. Let your walking or dance steps be lifted by a profound hope, love, or desire. Make your new job or career a work of joy. All these creative acts reveal who you are—there is no "wrong" way. Take the solo— move further along your own path, back to the garden. Find that place again of comfort and joy. Paint with your words, dance, or music—reveal the colors, sounds, and movements of your inmost being. Like Herman Hesse's Sinclair, let your creativity direct you back to the garden—to the paradise you have always known and where you find the source of your true self.

FIVE — SUPPORTING CAST AND SURROUNDING CHARACTERS: KITH AND KIN

Of the many comedians of the last century, George Burns was one of the greatest. He felt everyone could benefit from laughter and approached making people laugh as an art. Living to be 100 years old, he was renowned for telling jokes about getting older.[1] He often made light of the challenges encountered with advancing age, constructing jokes like, "You know you're getting older when... your favorite news section is 'What happened Fifty Years ago!' " Or, "...when an exciting Friday Night activity with friends is comparing your Advance Medical Directives!" Apart from helping us to laugh, and often to laugh at ourselves, comedy serves as a defense mechanism that allows us to look beyond the difficult circumstances we may be facing. Our attempts to find humor in our living also reveals something else about us—it tells us about our creativity, our current and past life-experiences and concerns, reflects our culture, and mirrors our worldview.[2] Moreover, humor also communicates what is possible through its wordplay and the imaginative concepts it conveys. Sometimes a joke emphasizes the tension between opposites and suggests commonalities that might be considered—like the "A priest, a rabbi and an atheist walk into a bar..." type of joke. A joke may also provide an insight into how we might look at life, and how we may care about and help each other. We also recognize that humor may be found in unlikely places. For example, while laughter is a unique characteristic of humans, it has been suggested that dogs may laugh too![3] Thus, considering the African proverb, "The dog never minds not to laugh," we note the strong bond between humans and dogs, and how we often use humor to face challenging life circumstances, and perhaps, realize that the dog is always keen to laugh with us—not at us! This connection between humor, ourselves, and our pets is exemplified in cartoons such as Garfield, Calvin and Hobbes, and Marmaduke, that many enjoy reading.

71

Humor also creates a social atmosphere and tells us about our family. One author had a wonderful Uncle George (not named Burns) who was always ready with a funny joke or a light-hearted way of looking at life. He reminded us of our human potential to overcome by making light of the situation and embracing a hope for better things in the future. He had confronted many life-challenges, yet was known for his resolve not to dwell on the negative aspects of the current trial or tribulation. His joyful demeanor, optimistic attitude, calmness in the moment and resolve, was uplifting for all those around him. Facing various existential crises, we often become aware of and discover the great personal strength and resources we possess, as we share our concerns with close confidants, family, and friends. Indeed, the emotional and practical support we receive from and in-turn give to those dearest to us, to friends, and to others in our community promotes an *esprit de corps*—a sense of closeness, common understanding, and loyalty, that offers moral support and real-world assistance, and serves as a powerful motivation to overcome life's challenges. We realize too that we are not alone. Others have met with and endured similar challenges. As we embrace our kith and kin, we draw upon a vast collection of personalities and styles of coping, common experiences, and deeply held beliefs and values that have a powerful influence on our thoughts, feelings, and actions. Thus, the appropriate sharing of one's humor and resilient attitude during times of challenge has a profound effect on how others may understand the moment and continue in their living, adaptively. In the case of the joking uncle, it was reported that he laughed when he received the absurd "Get Well" card as he faced terminal cancer. His light-heartedness and hope-filled attitude, always reassuring, continues to be inspirational to those who knew him. Another example is that of an older brother who, with the steel of a U.S. Marine, expressed a buoyant attitude throughout a long and final battle with illness. In his familiar way, weakened but still of irrepressible spirit the evening he died, he offered a smile and wink goodnight for the last time. Letting others know of his deep love and care for them, and his attitude of jest and bravery as death approached. Thus, laughter is a way of coping, of healing, and of promoting unity. The artful use of humor may be an aspect of our resilient attitude. It may also be one of those essential and defining characteristics of our personality, and something we inherit biologically and will pass on to our families. In effect then, humor is found in all cultures and is an implicit feature that affects our relationships with family and friends. Thus, humor is a social "art," and contributes to other social arts that allow us to live harmoniously with others, and that aid us in our journey to live authentically.

Cultural Backdrop

As we consider families and communities, we note the various cultural worldviews and life-values they promote. A worldview suggests specific ways of looking at life and understanding the world in which we live. In many ways then, our cultural context imposes and serves as a kind of perceptual filter that sets the stage for how we see the world and how we live in it. Our culture directs and inspires our imagination and creativity, and designates what we hold sacred and how we see others in relation to ourselves. Moreover, our worldview reflects the archetypal personas and stories of our culture. Like great works of art, these personas and stories reveal our deepest held concerns and communicate ways of living and being in the world. As the social psychologist Geert Hofestede and colleagues have suggested, these unwritten social practices and cultural norms are the "software of the mind."[4] Further, while reflecting diverse lifestyles and ways of thinking, worldviews often express the universal values of being trustworthy and honoring commitments, telling the truth, caring for others, protecting those who are vulnerable, and being loyal to family, clan, or community.[5]

Richly Brocaded Worldviews

As we consider worldviews and universal values, we might say that cultures are all relatively alike in some ways. After all, we are all human, and have similar concerns for our survival, family care, fairness in relationships, involvement and responsibility within communities, and ways of "knowing" ourselves. But if we look closer, we do see richly woven frameworks that are varied. For example, differences between the me-first, or individualistic, and us-together, or collectivist societies, or between the different expressions of spiritual or religious faiths and their respective transcendental concerns and ideologies are dimensions that we see represented within various worldviews. One pattern of variation is in the contrast between individualism and collectivism found respectively in Western versus Eastern societies. For example, those of us in the West are likely to view the world as comprised of individual objects, rather than as entities that are related to one another and form a conceptual whole.[6] This mindset leads to a self-aggrandizing and ego-centric orientation, where we are culturally predisposed to express our independence and uniqueness, as opposed to seeing ourselves in a broader context where we live interdependently and in relation with others. Comedic satire helps to elucidate these cultural moorings, as well as the possible ills they may produce. For example, Norman Lear's *All in the Family* and *The Jeffersons* situational comedies from the 1970's and 1980s (and still playing in reruns), respectively featuring the protagonists Archie Bunker and George Jefferson and their families, keenly represent western culture expressions of individualism, competition, and materialism, while also exposing the social problems of racism, sexism, and ageism.[7] Other more contemporary situational comedies like Kenya Barris' *Blackish*, and Steven Levitan and Christopher Lloyd's *Modern Family* re-boot these themes, adding the perspectives and concerns of feminism, gender identity, black culture, gay parenting, blended families, police brutality, and sexual expression.[8] The great value of these and other satirical works is that through their engaging humor and dramatic expression, they bring to light the deeper tensions and biases of our unconscious mind, allowing us to know ourselves better. As a result then, we may find ways to improve our relationships within our families and others in our community. Thus, finding a way to work with what may be uneasy and difficult topics for some, comedic satire often helps us to address various malignant characteristics that keep us from seeing others like ourselves and growing as a person.

Looking within the Eastern worldview, we find reflections of the centuries-old cultural traditions of Buddhism, Taoism, and Confucianism. These traditions promote and foster a social welfare that emphasizes respect for elders (filial piety) and the cultivation of compassion, cooperation, and moral enlightenment as key features and characteristics of the honorable person. Further, in comparison to the Western cultural perspective, the Eastern worldview is collectivist in orientation, rather than individualistic, and emphasizes interdependency among group members. Thus, identity is defined through loyal membership and cooperative group or organizational involvement. A dramatic expression of this worldview is noted in ancient stories revised for modern films and television programs featuring superheroes like the characters Guan Yin (also called Kuan Yin) and Sun Wukong (the Monkey King) from the pantheon of gods and goddesses noted in ancient Chinese mythology.[9] While these ancestral stories reflect a cultural orientation of interdependence, cooperation, and non-materialism, they also like the western worldview depict and characterize negative aspects of the human condition. For example, the story of Guan Yin, the dutiful daughter of a Chinese emperor, seeking to live a monastic life suffers the maltreatment and persecution of her all-controlling and tyrannical father. Nevertheless, Guan Yin miraculously endures the many schemes of her father to do away with her. Ultimately, through her great virtue she ascends to heaven, and later, as her father becomes ill, becomes his rescuer. Constant throughout Guan Yin's story is her expression of piety and love. Thus, she is celebrated as the goddess of Compassion and Mercy. Another ancient story involves the rather comical Sun Wukong, the Monkey god, who is sent by Guan Yin to retrieve the sacred scriptures that have been carried off to a far-away land. In this story, Sun Wukong's all too human hope for immortality, and playful and self-indulgent nature are revealed. But beyond his apparent mischievous and narcissistic characteristics, he also demonstrates heroic capabilities that allow him to return with the sacred works, and thus also becomes revered and celebrated as a god.[10] In both of these stories, we respectively find expression of moral excellence and virtuous living that leads to the purest joy and happiness, as well as the pratfall and slap-stick comedy of our own self-deceptions and egocentricities.

Other worldviews also embody and stress a communal orientation. For example, Indigenous and First Nations People throughout the world hold to their unique cultural traditions and customs, yet express a universalism that emphasizes a oneness and connection with the natural world and all forms of life. Further, there is a noted connection to place and community that highlights responsibility to care for the environment and one another. From this holistic perspective, human development is envisaged as a circle of life, moving from birth to death in a way that is interconnected and experienced with other creatures and all the universe. Thus, the cultural frameworks of Indigenous and First Nations People place importance on the sacredness of place, mystical relationship to the earth and its inhabitants, and the importance of values and morals for living. These earliest frameworks for living proclaim an oral tradition that celebrates communal knowledge and ways of understanding the world, and often incorporates a long history of cultural oppression. The illustrious power of laughter to express a connection to community, to build bridges, and to heal, is also celebrated in the oral traditions and contemporary cultural films, novels, and other creative works of these communities. Humor's ability to bring light to difficult topics and key cultural concerns helps in finding remedies to the many problems faced by indigenous communities.[11] Yet, these concerns, often offered with comedic bombast and accompanied by the audience's nervous laughter, likewise expose and make us aware of the not so funny undertones of racial and ethnic prejudices, cultural genocides, and discriminations and unresolved inequities that still continue.

Another worldview to note is found within Sub-Saharan Africa societies that practice the tradition of communitarianism.[12] The concept of communitarianism suggests that each person optimally develops through the support and molding of the community. Thus, the axiom of the Igbo and Yoruba tribes, "It takes a village to raise a child," is illustrative of a worldview that emphasizes shared responsibility, with a distinct focus on honoring communal traditions and living in harmony. From this orientation an obligation to be compassionate and caring towards others is inculcated, so that connection with and being part of the broader community becomes the central aspect of one's identity. As recognized in films and literature that reflect the many existential challenges that have befallen African societies in the modern era, this community-centric orientation seeks to value, care for, and protect each person within the community.[13] Again, as we find within all cultures, humor is used as a way of seeing the "big-picture," and navigating to a point of view that is restorative, and that may bring forth opportunity for social change, communal healing, and peace.[14] As sociologist and international relations scholar Ebenezer Obadare suggests, in doing so, the humor may be both self-deprecating and a criticism of the state.[15] Embracing communitarianism then, we may reflexively laugh knowing how much more affluent countries and wealthy corporations must do to end the exploitive practices of colonialism, restore just and equitable relations between nations, and work to see all persons, young and old, and their cultural community as equals. Furthermore, while some might continue to laugh and say that will never happen, revealing the uneasy tension of our hidden biases, it may be only through humor, perhaps, that we may begin to address and resolve the many current social injustices that afflict communities throughout the world.

We are cast in many roles in life. Our worldview, like a theatre stage backdrop, reflects unique cultural features that affect how we relate to and interact with members of our families, people with whom we work or volunteer, and others throughout the broader communities in which we reside. Our life in many ways is an ongoing drama, often filled with an anxiousness as we grapple with the challenges that involve our interactions with others and important societal concerns. The climax and ultimate relief in this drama will demand that we discover new ways of meeting and working with these challenges, while still being true to self and supportive of our community. Laughter can be an elixir for whatever ails us, and a tool that may help us reframe life-concerns in a way that aids our personal growth and connection with others. Our ability to laugh, discover new ways of coping, and to come to the aid of others is perhaps at its peak in the second half of the life-course, when we are more able to weigh the ultimate value and meaning of our lives, and recognize the importance of our contribution to family and community.

Kith and Kin

Through our families we learn a basic sense of trust and interdependence, and ways of communicating and interacting in relationships. In all cultural settings, we become aware of our shared interests and sense that we "belong" to each other. Thus, based on our individual needs and personal characteristics, we express and provide care and support for one another. Yet, within the family, everyone may communicate this care and support in a different way. For example, we may feel a closeness to one or both parents, or to a sibling, so that there is a rather congenial relationship, with relatively high levels of involvement in life activities, and few areas or topics where there is discontent or jealousy. However, relationships are complicated. Common interests and shared successes in some areas are celebrated, whereas resentments and envy may also be present—especially when we consider the complex dynamics of parent-child and sibling relationships. This reality is expressed in a very humorous way by the musical and comedic duo the Smothers Brothers from the 1960s (a touring act until Tom's death in 2023), revealing a universal concern that tells us we are always in the process of "working out the details" of our relationships. In their stage act, the Smothers Brothers portrayed this relational antipathy and longstanding grievance, with Tommy reporting to brother Dick that, "Mom always liked you best!" Other contemporary situational comedies like the *Goldbergs* also remind us of the different parenting styles children may receive, from the over-protective and smothering to the emotionally detached, as well as the rivalries that may exist between siblings.[16] Thus, while family relations are often thought to be loving and supportive, they may also be lacking in closeness, involvement, and contact, and feel suffocating as patterns of hostility, resentments and envy endure. Further, while ties between siblings are suggested to be closest during adolescence and again later in life, due to evolving cultural values and demands of caregiving, research suggests that at midlife not all siblings may offer or provide care to aging parents.[17] Thus, in the middle of life, how we may be caregivers both to children as well as for aging parents, and how we might fulfill these roles are again influenced by our own personal needs and characteristics.

A sense of responsibility to take care of one another and the provision of mutual aid are often motivating factors underlying the older parent-adult child relationship. In fact, many older parents still offer all the economic, moral, and emotional assistance to their children that they can. In a reciprocal way, adult children often offer support and assistance to older parents who face poor health and/or deteriorating financial conditions. Nevertheless, we recognize the evolving patterns and diverse qualities of intergenerational relationships. For example, parents and adult children may express a politic of the earlier child-parent relationship, where parents are still in charge and children should obey. But as we grow into adulthood and into later life, we can form new relationships with our parents and children. In addition, in later life, the liberation from child rearing responsibilities, along with increased personal freedom and privacy, provides new opportunities for the older adult to explore their own interests. This liberation often leads to an enhancement of personal well-being. Thus, in later life parents and children often express positive feelings for one another, as the elder, feeling a closeness, sees the child as a friend and confidant.

As we broaden consideration of relationships, we recognize extensive kinship ties. These family ties may be simple, focusing just on parents and children. They may also be more expansive, involving several generations and a blending of family members that include siblings and intimate connections that may extend beyond the boundaries of our genetic family tree. Thus, kinship includes parents and children, as well as grandparents and other relatives and associates that are regarded as "family." As previously noted, at midlife, we may find ourselves playing the role of helping children transition into their own adult lives (e.g., moving out of the home, starting jobs, creating families), as well as taking care of aging parents, grandparents, and other older family members. We may also be cast in the new role of being a grandparent. All these roles suggest ways we are kith and kin keepers within our families, and that may offer wonderful fulfillments or impose steep demands requiring some manner of personal adjustment.

Certainly, one may feel a heightened sense to take care of parents and grandparents at midlife. The term filial obligation refers to this sense of responsibility to care for one's parents. When we think about caring for an elderly parent, we should be aware that family members, including children, provide most of the support and day-to-day care needed. Concomitant with roles designated via one's cultural worldview, however, daughters most often are the ones who coordinate and provide most of the care for elderly parents. Without a doubt, caregiving can be a trying task. It is noted that caregivers are 3 to 4 times more likely than non-caregivers to report symptoms of depression and anger.[18] Thus, it should be noted that the respective stress and rewards of caregiving are many. Some of the negative outcomes include resentment for being cast in the caregiving role; anger directed at parents, siblings, or self; feelings of being overloaded or feeling guilty in some way; and feeling burned-out; along with the exacerbation of risk for impaired physical and mental health; and potential for taking on new financial burdens. Some of the positive outcomes, however, include a sense of fulfilling family obligations; spending time together and having moments of enjoyment and laughter; and knowing the individual is being well cared for.[19]

Grandparenting

Other kith and kin relationships include grandparent and grandchildren connections. There are a several ways of grandparenting, ranging from playing a more traditional role, to the active and fun-loving, to the more distant and remote, and substitute- or surrogate-parent involvements.[20] All of these approaches offer opportunities to share one's creative ideas and expression.[21] For example, in the more traditional role, the grandparent is occasionally involved with grandchildren in indulging activities and baby-sitting, but does not serve in the "real" practice of parenting. Here we might recognize the passing on of family stories, rife with archetypal characters such as sage, hero, and magician, as an example of imaginative and creative expression exchanged between grandparents and grandchildren. Another type of grandparenting is one oriented around having fun, and typifies an energetic and young-at-heart grandparent who involves the grandchild in fun activities. In this orientation there may be special focus on passing on one's passion for joyful living or in using humor to suggest a happy way to live life, characterized through all manner of creative activity and expression. Another type of grandparenting is where due to distance between families, or because of illness, contact with grandchildren is limited, and only the occasional exchange of things like gifts and cards may occur. Even with reduced contact, however, we may still see a sharing of artistic interests and a passing down of one's imaginative approach or tools for creative expression. But when illness or dramatic changes in the grandparent's intellectual or physical functioning occur, children may especially feel a loss of the grandparent, even though they continue living. Indeed, as a 12-year-old visitor to one of the author's classrooms starkly remarked concerning changes in personality and cognitive functioning that he observed in his grandmother following a major stroke: "She wasn't my grandma anymore!"

Another type of grandparenting is where the older person takes on the child-rearing role, either part-time (e.g., for working mothers) or full-time (e.g., for parents who are not able to take care of children for some reason). Cast in the role of surrogate-parent, these grandparents assist the grandchild in enrollment in school, receiving health care, and providing the grandchild with a place to live. With the burden of raising another child later in life, these older substitute-parents experience more stress and disruption of everyday roles than traditional grandparents. Nevertheless, the whole creative palette remains available to use in sharing one's imaginative and artistic interests. In this substitute-parenting role, certainly the elder is cast as leading actor and authority within the family structure, but also serves as key dispenser of support, love, and family wisdom. It should also be noted that divorce may disrupt the contact grandparents have with grandchildren. Thus, contact between grandparents and grandchildren may vary as a function of which parent has custody of or residential arrangement for the child.[22]

Being a great-grandparent is another role one may play in later life, and represents a time where the older individual may undergo a personal renewal as they sense an extending of the generations, or feel a change in one's life journey. As a great-grandparent, one may continue to share one's wisdom and vast repertoire of experience, as well as all of one's imagination and creativity with grandchildren.[23] Moreover, great-grandparenting may be a time when one feels more inclined to express through their storytelling or other creative expressions how one might live honorably, morally, and successfully adapt to life's challenges.[24]

Friends and Lovers: There Is an Art to All of This Too!

As suggested by the famous psychiatrist Erich Fromm, loving is an art. Thus, like other arts we can grow in our understanding of its many different dimensions and expressions, and learn how to best practice it in our everyday living.[25] Further, as a recent survey suggests, loving and feeling loved are very important concerns for most of us in later life.[26] Yet, this is another complicated area, and reflects the difficulties it presents when we hear someone say: "Love... it only hurts when I laugh!" Certainly, the depth and enduring strength of our love relationships is often contingent on our developing a sense of trust with the other person, so that we may share our deepest and most intimate feelings and concerns. As we alluded earlier, this is not a simple task for many of us. Moreover, as younger or older adults, we may have different love expectations or needs that we hope the intimate other will help us attain. Indeed, research in this area suggests that the nature of love is characterized differently by younger and older adults, with older lovers emphasizing the importance of emotional security and loyalty, with sexual intimacy being of lesser importance.[27] Yet, we all want to be loved, and romances and love affairs in later life do occur, with or without the expression of tender feelings, a sense of deep sharing or intimacy, or feelings of compatibility. As Robert Sternberg proposes, the interpersonal relationship we call "love" involves a story we tell about ourselves and share with another.[28] Accordingly, when we find a person who fits with the roles and attributes of our love story, we may form a loving relationship with them. Moreover, the more closely the other is matched to the ideal attributes and roles within our love story, the more satisfying the relationship.[29] Again, this love story and the partner's matching of attributes and roles is complex. Thus, at any age, forming a loving relationship presents many challenges, including how to form a loving relationship free of illusions, how to maintain one's sense of autonomy, and how to find a supportive emotional balance in the relationship.[30] Some of the most enduring love relationships start out as friendships. Love relationships that have spanned many years are often described as continuing in this friendship, companionship, and romance.

Friends are important sources of emotional, moral, and practical support throughout life. In general, we may enjoy intimate, deeply emotional, and confiding types of friendships, as well as friendships that are less intimate and involve some type of competitiveness. Yet, as we advance into later life it is not uncommon to see a reduction in the number of people that we remain in contact or become involved with as we get older. When we consider the number of people that make up our social network then, we are likely to count fewer older family members, friends, and casual contacts with advancing age. For most of us, our social networks are probably their largest during our school years (i.e., adolescence and young adulthood). But as we begin careers and start our own families, we are often less likely to maintain contact with all our peers and friends from earlier times in life. Therefore, in midlife, social networks typically involve family members and very close friends. This decline continues into older age where we may lose parents and siblings as well as spouses or partners.

Surely, a richness can be found in the relationships we form with others throughout our lives. As we reflect, we may sense an understanding of how we have benefited or have been challenged and have grown as a result of particular friendships or relationships. When we consider our continued development into older age, we become aware of the many different social roles we have played or will play in life and confront the loss of family members and close friends. For many of us, the most significant losses we experience as we journey into midlife and older age are the loss of grandparents, parents, brothers and sisters, spouses, and partners. While we may always remember their joking manner and miss their laughter, in the changes and losses we encounter there is a hope we will find yet new insights and understandings into our current relationships.

Other "Social" Arts and Finding Wholeness

Perhaps one of the most basic ways we tell someone we care about them is through sharing a meal with them. Indeed, as noted in a life story interview from one of the authors' Life Story Project, sharing food is a symbolic way of celebrating life and expressing our care for those we love.[31] But life isn't always easy, and we learn more about life through the arts of compromise and cooperation. As one retired teacher and guest to one author's college classroom noted, sometimes we come to a turning point when we realize we must find a way to change how we understand and relate to one another. Discussing his "old-school methods" to control an unruly classroom, the retired teacher was asked, "When did you come to a turning point?" Without skipping a beat, he shrugged and said, "When I was berating my son for only getting Cs on his grade report from college, and my son calmly but assertively said: 'Dad, I have feelings too!' " At that moment he related he realized his yelling and scathing comments were not building closeness, nor offering support. We must give and take in our relationships, and struggle to work out all the little details. Thus, perhaps the greatest challenge we will face is building satisfying relationships with those we love and those we encounter in our life. But again, it isn't easy. The following interviews from the Life Story Project conducted by one of the authors help us understand these challenges. Describing early times of life, adverse childhood events, and difficult times in their marriages, careers, and volunteering experiences, as well as their philosophy for living, and the role of humor and times of happiness in their lives, K.H. and D.S. share their stories.[32]

K.H.'s Story

I was the first-born in a family of three children, and we lived in a home that my dad's mom owned. Looking back, we were lower-middle class and I think we got along well. We had food on the table, but we were by no means wealthy. We played outside and made lots of friends with the neighborhood kids, and we played games like kick-the-can and hide-and-seek. We went home when we were hungry, and if we weren't we'd just play all day. At that time, I don't think anyone had a concern for bad things that could happen to children. It was very different. My sisters and I were the three musketeers. We'd do a lot of things together and had a lot of mutual friends.

In the sixth grade, I sort of became the nerd of the family. This could have been because I was being bullied. There was kind of a "gang" in our neighborhood, with a bunch of tough kids. They would go after me. When we would go ice skating in the winter, if those boys were there, they would throw me in the snowbanks and threaten to beat me up. I became rather reclusive because of that, and I would hide out at the house. When I saw them in the streets I would run because I was really afraid, even when walking to and from school. I always had to watch out for those guys. I lived in a state of fear. I didn't feel good about it. I felt insecure and was watching my back at all times. I couldn't be myself. Part of the reason I decided to go to a private boy's school was to avoid those bully guys and their harm.

At one point in high school, I fell in love with my best friend. The worst part of it was that I knew he was not gay. I was about 17 years old, and I tried to commit suicide. I took a bottle of sleeping pills. With the help of my therapist, at the age of 24, I came to terms with who I was, and was able to accept myself. Later, when I met my husband, the adoption of our sons, and birth of my grandson, those were the happiest times of life. Life events like that, where I was interacting with other people and sharing events with others made me the happiest. Later we became separated, and my husband committed suicide. That was very difficult.

My philosophy for living is primarily being good, and being good to each other by helping each other, and doing what you can for others. I hold the belief that others will treat you well if you follow this philosophy... I find happiness by being very optimistic, by finding humor in a lot of things. Like even in the class on cremation I attended recently, that you would think would be a serious class. But during the class I sat and joked with my classmates and had a good discussion. I find a lot of humor in various situations, joking with people and talking with people. Also, in giving of myself. Last night I volunteered four hours at the hospital rocking babies and that makes me happy. I also enjoy spending time with my grandson. He is five years old and pretends to be a superhero, and we play in the basement, and that makes me happy.

In another interview, D.S. shares about her early experiences and life journey, expressing ways of overcoming challenges and making compromises, and in later life always wanting to have fun.

D.S.'s Story

I was born near the Detroit area... an only child and grew up in a neighborhood where my grandmother lived across the street from me. My parents both worked, and every morning I went to my grandmother's house to finish getting ready to go to school. It was when we could still walk to school, walk home for lunch, and go back to school.

Everything was within walking distance. My father was gone for WWII, and it was hard for my mom and me. But my grandparents were always there for me. When I was eight years old my father came back. He got a new job... working in North Carolina. This was different because we had always lived close to all our family. We were only there for a little while due to my father dying in a plane crash. The radio announced it before they even told us. This was a pretty traumatic experience, especially hearing it on the radio first.

When we moved back, my mother remarried and lived in Dearborn, Michigan. In middle school and high school there was nothing I really liked about the kids. Everything was cliquey-cliquey-cliquey. Most of my friends were college bound, and once I got to college, I absolutely loved it. I was living in a dorm and had all these sisters and joined a sorority. I got my degree as a teacher and it was an easier time. I taught for 20 years in the same school... then got my master's degree and got married. Soon after, my husband got a job in Chicago, and as we made this transition, I decided I did not want to teach in Chicago.

After we moved to Chicago we had some marriage problems and divorced. I needed to find a job, so I recreated my resume so that it didn't seem like the only thing I had ever done in my life was teach. Unknowingly, I ran into a really nice fellow who was able to find me a job in technology training for Macintosh computers. I ended up being a regional sales manager, even though I did not know anything about marketing. I began to work for Apple under Steve Jobs, and I got to preview all the projects that rolled out before they were sold to the public. The divorce was easy because I was preoccupied with my friends, and I was traveling four out of five days of the week. I was comfortable with the new lifestyle.

After the divorce, I ran into a new gentleman after some time. He was a lawyer and owned a restaurant in Chicago. There were red flags all over that relationship that

I chose to ignore. The big flags were that he did not respect my things at my house. He also had a special needs child. I had great hopes that I would be able to move mountains and help with her education, as I had been a very good teacher. I found myself losing myself. My friends would ask me what was wrong with me. None of my friends liked this new man in my life. Well, I had bought a house for his daughter so she could receive additional care through a special needs program. So, there was an extra house. I started to furnish it, and little by little I had my getaway house. When I left him, I had a place to go. When living alone, I had my mom, so I was not alone.

Living independently, I started to find volunteer work because it was fun, and it was a great way to pass time. I did not want to teach again but I helped in the classrooms. I work at an elementary school in a mentoring program, and that is fun. I am very happy with my lifestyle. Even now, I look at my house and ask myself if I should clean the house or go have fun elsewhere. I always go have fun. I am 80 years old, and I love dancing. I drive and I don't have any health issues.

In both K.H. and D.S.'s stories we hear of the joys of earlier times, as well as traumatic experiences and the many challenges that arise as we grow up and mature. As Erik Erikson and Irvin Yalom have instructed,[33] these early traumatic events continue to be a part of our life story, and thus may reappear in some manner in our thinking and acting later in life and require redress to find closure and healing so that one can move past them and live adaptively. Thus, in their stories we find universal concerns for one's personal safety, sense of security, forming an identity, and the ongoing pursuit to find happiness and its realization in the loving and joy-filled associations we form with family and friends. As we consider life stories that tell of great challenges and moments of happiness, we want to share one more that emphasizes the arts of embracing transition and finding wholeness. It is found in the story of Father

Joseph Champlin, a Catholic priest living in Camillus, New York, and his battle with cancer throughout his 70s.

From Wellness to Illness and Back

As one of the authors met with Father Champlin, a prolific writer and gifted speaker on issues of faith and relationships, he did not talk about his life and tell of his story, but rather simply provided a copy of his latest book, *From Time to Eternity and Back: A Priest's Successful Struggle with Cancer*.[34] In this autobiographical work, Father Champlin discusses his journey from wellness to illness and back again, as he battles Waldenstrom's Macroglobulinemia, a type of non-Hodgkin lymphoma (NHL). First diagnosed in his early 70s, he describes the uncertainty of survival, the anxiety associated with diagnosis and the difficulties of chemotherapy, as well as the discovery of an outpouring of support, care, and love from friends and others in his community. Waldenstrom's Macroglobulinemia is a cancer that first begins in the white blood cells, and may cause a variety of effects including bleeding of the nose or gums, easy bruising, fatigue, difficulty breathing, fever, headache, and confusion. As Father Champlin writes, waiting for the diagnosis and wondering what will happen next wasn't easy. Many readers may know the tormenting anxiety associated with waiting for illness confirmation—our thoughts and emotions tend to race in a wild torrent until we receive information that reduces our uncertainty and shows us the next mountain we will be asked to climb. In Father Champlin's case the next mountain was the battle to survive chemotherapy.

Providing a blow-by-blow description of his battle with cancer, Father Champlin dramatically details the disruptions to everyday life, rounds of nausea that accompany chemotherapy, and loss of mental and physical strength that leads one to feel like they are "out-on-their-feet." The good news is that this type of cancer can be treated and managed. However, it would still be a chronic health problem that Father Champlin would always have to contend with and shorten his life. In his story we come to sense and understand the adage, "if the disease doesn't kill you—sometimes the cure will." Yet, Father Champlin did survive the treatment, and slowly recovered his strength to live in remission with this rather rare form of cancer.

As Father Champlin's story suggests, we can learn a great deal from the various crises we face in life. What he reported to be the most remarkable were the many gifts and messages of support and love provided by others, and the inner strength that he did not know he would discover during his illness. Father Champlin's story portrays the inevitability of a critical and no holds barred life-review—a looking back, but also a looking ahead into whatever shadowy abyss or illuminated paradise or nothingness we might imagine. In his journey from wellness to illness and back again, he remarked that his road to recovery was the same as that travelled by those who suffer addiction or other chronic illnesses. It is a road where fellow travelers share the same plaintive hope and pray for a greater power to provide relief, to give insight and aid in finding deeper meaning, and to offer deliverance into a new wholeness beyond the illness experience. As Father Champlin offers, and as K.H. and D.S. also implicitly suggest in their stories, he learned the sorrow and pain of loss, greater appreciation for the moments of happiness and for all the things held dear. He grasped anew the humbleness of one's good works, and the enormous and enduring love others bestow on us. His story is one of a conversion into a deeper faith and trust, and a more profound awareness of the love that we receive and that we may give until the very last moment of our life. Father Champlin survived another seven years after his first diagnosis of cancer and died at 77 years of age.

Don't Forget the Dog!

We should also mention how endeared pets and other animals may assist us and be a source of comfort. Certainly, as we tend to the needs of our pets, things like feeding the goldfish, misting the soil of our pet beetle's terrarium, and walking the family dog, we recognize how indispensable we are in providing for their care. In their special way too, through tail wags, "licks and kisses" and purrs of contentment, family pets may express and provide us a strong sense of feeling needed, being appreciated, and having a purpose in our living. Beyond helping to fulfill these basic psychological needs, the comfort and warmth of a pet may also provide physical health benefits. For example, as noted in several research reviews, petting and holding a dog or cat has been suggested to lower cognitive and attendant physiological stress.[35] Moreover, owning a dog has been found to be associated with lower blood pressure, cholesterol levels and plasma triglycerides; suggesting that the comfort of fido may help to reduce risk for heart disease and the management of other illnesses. Further, the presence of a therapy dog has been suggested to lower levels of anxiety, enhance communication and group cohesion in patients with chemical dependency, and provide comfort and reduce stigma for psychiatric patients as the dog expresses to the individual an unconditional acceptance. Pet ownership may also significantly increase life-satisfaction, reduce use of pain medications, serve as an aid to exercise routines (e.g., taking the dog for a walk), and provide practical assistance along with socio-emotional support.[36] Thus, as many pet owners remark, the family pet literally "gives me a reason to get out of bed in the morning!" So, it is easy to understand how and why we might find an intersection involving people, animals, and the arts. Indeed, there is a wide range of inspired songs about, *Me and You and a Dog named Boo,* and horses and cats and pets of all sorts, that portray this connection between humans, animals, and music.[37] One special case of this human-animal-music intersection to consider is that of Dr. Milton H. Dunsky, formerly Chief of Nuclear Medicine at the Veterans Administration Hospital and Department of Medicine at Upstate Medical Center in Syracuse, New York.[38]

Born in New York City to immigrant parents from Sulwalki, Poland, Dr. Dunsky took violin lessons during elementary school that established a foundation for his life-long love of music. Subsequent developmental influences included coming of age at the same time as the great jazz artists Dizzy Gillespie and Charlie Parker, and the heralded symphony director and *West Side Story* composer Leonard Bernstein's debut with the New York Philharmonic.[39] A jazz and classical music aficionado, Milton frequently played Stan Getz and Charlie Byrd's *Jazz Samba* album at dinner parties and various symphony recordings during family gatherings.[40] In his adult life, Milton was noted for always having a good story to tell, and a kind word to share. In performing his professional duties, Dr. Dunsky was known for his compassionate and conscientious practice of medicine, and a pleasant and unflappable concern for patients and students. Beyond his devotion to his family and passion for music, and in his caring style of living, another love of Dr. Dunsky was dachshunds. And over the many years, the family's dachshund-in-resident, affectionately named "Apples J. Puppydog," and later "Holly," "Hannah," and "Freddy," was a significant actor in the household scene. The family hound, when not sitting closely-at-foot under the dinner table awaiting special treats, would often prod her or his way onto the lap of daughter Mary Elizabeth during her piano practice, or onto Milton's lap while he listened to jazz and classical music recordings. Milton's love of music and of his dog was so great that often before the family left home to go on a short afternoon trip, he would turn on the classical music radio station so that symphonies by Berlioz, Beethoven, Brahms, and Mahler filled the air; much to the contentment and comfort of his beloved pet, who awaited loyally for the return of Dr. Dunsky, "Dog's best friend!"

How music further becomes part of the human-animal bond is suggested in an interview with Robert Dunsky, Milton's son, who remarks:

> I think that Dad would leave the music on for the dog because Dad superimposed humanness onto each of the dogs. If Dad were home alone, he would play the music for himself. Just the same, there are likely commonalities between the soothing effects of pet ownership and of listening to music. The common part might be the interactive component of music: Think playing "Air Drums," or swaying to a predictable beat, and interactions between the pet and owner. There is also the human-social component of pet ownership, like going to dog parks, meeting people while walking, attending outdoor music concerts with one's pet, and engaging in "pet-friendly"

discussion boards. Pet's and music bring people together and form a one-on-one bond. [41]

Later in life, when Milton suffered the ravages of motor-neuron disease and associated cognitive declines, Freddy, the family dachshund, remained a constant and comforting friend. Indifferent to Milton's physical and cognitive declines, Freddy, like the proverb noted at the beginning of this chapter, never minded not to laugh. He remained a faithful companion. Providing unconditional love and respect and communicating through his nuzzling and nudging to be upon Milton's lap, or in attendance nearby under his hospital bed — "I am here and will be with you, so let the music play on."

A Last Word — Remember to Laugh!

Some events in life are such that they cause us to laugh so hard that we are brought to tears. While other events are so tumultuous and difficult that they bring us to our knees in weeping despair, and we feel we will never laugh again. But indeed, we do laugh again, and we need to laugh. Throughout life laughter helps us learn about our need to love and care for one another, and to find compromise in our relationships. As we encounter changes in health, jobs, social and economic statuses, and loss of family members, laughter helps us become students of the arts of maintaining optimism, embracing transitions, and finding wholeness again. Laughter, through its enlivening and restorative balm, supports us as we venture forth in life. Indeed, humor and comedy are often an important element and composite of the creative roads we travel in becoming an authentic person and living to our fullest potential. So, let us not forget the importance of laughter. Thus, like the yester-year television entertainer Art Linkletter, and more recently comedian Tiffany Haddish, who ask kids what they think and how they see the world, we may be reminded of the great imaginative insight of childhood, and experience again the fun and laughter that children share — a laughter that in its hearing can make us whole again.[42] Further, as the writer Norman Cousins discovered, laughter may give us a new lease on life — providing such a powerful antidote to stress and enhancement of our immunological response when facing grave illness, that even death has to wait a while longer for the punch-line.[43] So remember to laugh—in the joyous guffaws and giggles we share, we become one. In our snicker, snorts, and belly laughs, we find relief from life-sorrows, pains, and illnesses, and begin to cross a bridge that offers a restorative healing for people from all backgrounds and from all places.

As Marcus Tullius Cicero wrote more than 2000 years ago, each moment in life has advantages and disadvantages.[1] Some of the advantages of later life include the gift of experience, knowledge, and wisdom. While in contrast, the disadvantages include declines in biophysical functioning and increased risk for disease and illness. We can also face an antagonist in our own self-appraisal, as we ask ourselves, "at my age, what can I still do physically and mentally?" The resulting self-evaluation may mirror back to us the negative stereotypes of older people expressed through various media, or the dread we might feel thinking we too may succumb to the illnesses or infirmities we have seen family and friends encounter. Certainly, the worry we may feel considering the disadvantages of growing older is enough to lose your head over; and by the way, that is how Marcus Tullius Cicero met his end — in the literal "cut-throat" political world of ancient Rome, as his rival, Mark Antony, declared Marcus an enemy of the state and ordered his assassination. In this chapter, with the hope that we will not come to such a gruesome ending, we will discuss changes in sensory-perceptual processes, physical functioning, and risk for disease, and also consider the stories of older adults that suggest ways in which our creative expressions can transport us into a joyful celebration of living.

Aging is a Natural Process

Aging is a natural, intrinsic, universal, and inevitable process. Nevertheless, "aging" is considered an undesirable term, that, with its intense focus on adverse changes and declines that may occur as we get older, has spurred the development of a multi-billion dollar industry proposing a wide array of antiaging therapies.[2] Further, holding close to this negative view of aging, one model of later life experience makes implicit connection between a variety of adverse health outcomes and existential disturbances that one may encounter.[3] This deficit-oriented model posits aging as a transition from a time of Independent Living, where one will likely lament the aches and pains of growing older, to a time of Interdependency, where one will have greater need for assistance from others, and require various accommodations (e.g., bath area grab bars and shower chairs, wheel-chair ramps, and health monitoring technology). Continuing this downward spiral, the model describes the next phase of later life as that of Dependency, where there will be a need to rely on others for transportation and assistance with other tasks of instrumental living (e.g., preparing food, banking, executive decision making). The final stages of the model construe life much like an ongoing series of health crises and medical emergencies and are thusly labelled Crisis Management and End-of-Life. This depersonalizing and stereotyped description of later life would seem to suggest that older adults are more of a burden needing to be "aided and managed" into the oblivion of their non-existence, rather than a great resource and rich treasure. In contrast, we have advocated that respecting and valuing each person and their lived experiences is crucial to our understanding of the diverse experiences of older people and later life. Moreover, we have submitted that through one's creative endeavors we enter onto the grand avenues, side-streets and footpaths leading us to new insights and ways of celebrating our life and that of others as we all get older. Thus, we have emphasized the importance of focusing on the relevant experiences and psychology of the individual, as depicted in their life stories and found in their artistic and creative expressions. From our perspective then, rather than a time of decline and despite the shifting statuses of health and well-being that occur throughout adulthood, we propose later life to be a time of many new possibilities and further growth as a person. Indeed, as we see the person mature, we witness the flourishing of interests and talents, and of a greater blossoming of the human spirit. However, we cannot simply ignore the physical and psychosocial changes that do occur as we get older. These changes are a real part of aging, and thus we propose that they also serve to help us discover and realize new meaning and purpose in our living. In the next sections, we look at changes in sensory-perceptual processes and physical health, and how these changes may impact our living.

Age-related Changes in Sensory-Perceptual Processes

With advancing age come changes in sensory-perceptual processes. These changes are significant because we come to know the world through our senses. Through our senses—vision, hearing, taste, touch, smell, and proprioception (as we dance for instance), we make manifest our desire to create. With vision, we recognize the gradual decline in the ability to focus on nearby objects, usually occurring after age 40.[4] Termed presbyopia, this is a common occurrence due to changes in the mechanical structures of the eye. For example, the lens of the eye, the peripheral visual mechanism that bends the light rays that pass through it in order to project a suitably sharp image on the retina, becomes thicker and less elastic, and more opaque as we age. These changes impact the ability of the lens to stretch and adjust focus (accommodate). Thus, static visual acuity, the ability to identify stationary objects (e.g., letters on the *Snellen Test*) declines markedly after age 45. With advancing age also comes yellowing of the lens. This change affects our color sensitivity, especially in the blue-green end of the spectrum. Other age-related changes include decline in pupil size that affects the amount of light reaching the retina and the need for brighter illumination to distinguish objects from a background. These changes are normal in the sense that they happen to most people as they get older. Yet, they affect our everyday experience and may impact upon creative activities like sewing, knitting, painting, drawing, or other arts that involve acute pattern recognition and spatial contrast to produce subtle nuance in design or other artistic expressions.

Beyond these normal age-related changes in vision, there are pathologic concerns as well. In fact, in the United States, eye disease affects 25% of those 80 years of age and older.[5] Cataracts, those cloudy or opaque areas that form on the lens of the eye, inhibiting the passage of light and causing a significant decline in vision, are a common eye disease in later life. Glaucoma and senile macular degeneration are also diseases of the eye that develop as the person ages. Glaucoma is an increase in fluid pressure in the eye that causes internal damage to the eye and results in loss of vision. Senile macular degeneration is also a problem that occurs when a specialized part of the retina responsible for reading and focusing on small details loses its ability to function effectively. For those who live with diabetes, diabetic retinopathy, the malfunction of small blood vessels that nourish the retina and causes damage that inhibits cellular functioning, may also impair vision. As these diseases impact our everyday living, they also negatively affect physical, cognitive, psychological, and social functioning, and are associated with greater prevalence of other chronic conditions (e.g., hypertension, heart disease, stroke, arthritis, chronic obstructive pulmonary disease, depression).[6] Thus, eye disease poses an existential threat as it may affect one's quality of life, as well as limit or curtail one's ability to participate in and enjoy self-expression through various creative activities. Accommodating tools for those with normal age-related changes in vision and low vision (i.e., where uncorrected vision in the best eye is less than 20/70 or poorer) include optical magnifiers, reading glasses, and telescopes for distal vision, as well as electronic magnifiers that can increase text or image size, or change the color-contrast of figural images and background on the page. Also available are low vision apps that magnify text and images, converts written text into spoken language, orients the person to aspects of the physical environment, monitors glucose levels, provides reminders when to take medicines, and arranges communication with health providers in the community.[7]

Our hearing also changes as we age, and decline in hearing sensitivity is the most prevalent sensory-perceptual loss.[8] For example, subtle, differential declines in sensitivity to the amplitude (i.e., loudness) and frequency (i.e., high or low pitch) of sound occur as we get older. That is, with advancing age we become less able to detect and thus hear high pitched sounds. This decline in sensitivity to high pitched sounds becomes more pronounced in frequencies above 12kHz. As a result, problems with speech perception also occur, as the consonants and vowels of language contain both high- and low-pitched sounds, making it more difficult to parse all the phonemic information (i.e., the sounds of language). Thus, as we noted regarding vision, with hearing we also see a rather common age-related decline. This is termed presbycusis and is a normal change in hearing caused by deterioration of mechanical structures of the ear over time. Yet, this decline may be exacerbated by chronic exposure to loud noises, use of certain drugs, improper diet, or genetic factors.

Again, like the area of vision, we also recognize pathologies that cause hearing loss. Hearing loss occurs when sound waves are unable to be transduced properly, caused by impediments in the ear such as dense wax, excessive fluid, abnormal bone growth, or the result of an infection that damages the cells of the inner ear. Auditory impairment caused by changes in neurological structures of the brain that process sound information may also occur, that resultantly affects one's ability to perceive sound or to understand language. Certainly, hearing loss presents many challenges for the person, and is suggested to cause communication dysfunction as well as loneliness, dependency, and frustration, all of which may diminish quality of life.[9] Hearing loss understandably poses a very great existential threat and significant life disruption for musicians. Preventing hearing loss includes turning the volume of radios, televisions, and amplifiers down, as well as avoiding places and activities that are noisy. Deterrence of hearing loss also includes using sound reducing earmuffs and earplugs, as well as sound shields. When hearing loss occurs, accommodating tools include sound augmenting devices like hearing aids, and, for profound hearing loss, cochlear implants that provide electrical stimulation of the auditory nerve through electrodes placed within the cochlea.

Other sensory-perceptual systems are also affected by aging. For most of us, changes in taste and smell occur as we get older, making detection of the sweet, bitter, sour, salty, and umami qualities of our taste sensations more difficult.[10] As a result, for those who express their creativity through the culinary arts, some foods prepared by older chefs may seem extra-spicy to a younger taster, due to a decline in the older chef's ability to detect the different spices and their adding more "to taste." Further, our ability to detect odors is best between ages 20 to 40, but begins to decline at age 50, and more rapidly after age 70. Thus, noted declines in the recognition and perceived intensity of odors occur in later life. Again, these changes are likely to affect the older culinary artists' craft, as well as the dining experience of the older individual, as smell is often part of the pleasure of our eating and drinking experience. As we similarly noted in the area of vision and hearing, decline in taste and smell detection may be associated with normal aging, but may be exacerbated in individuals with disease, or who use certain medications, or have been exposed to environmental pollutants, or have suffered neurological insult (e.g., traumatic brain injury), or from immunological assault to olfactory sensory neurons from contracting the Covid-19 virus.[11]

Touch, skin (temperature) and balance (proprioception) also change with advancing age.[12] For example, discrimination of distances between pressure administered to points on the skin, as well as the ability to identify objects through touch alone is also suggested to decline in older age. Further, with increasing age, vibratory stimulation of the skin surface is less easily detected, particularly in the lower extremities. Generally, temperature sensitivities and preferences do not differ between younger and older adults, but maintaining body temperature, and coping with cold and enduring hot environments are suggested to decline as we age.

The perception of acute pain, the unpleasant sensory and emotional experience associated with real or potential tissue damage, is associated with personality characteristics, thus the research on pain sensitivity is mixed, with some studies reporting a reduction in pain sensitivity with advancing age, while, others report no change, and others yet suggest an increase in pain sensitivity.[13] For chronic pain, however, the type that is persistent and localized in areas such as the back, joints, mouth, or face, is more often reported by older adults than by younger adults, and may be concomitantly associated with anxiety and depression.[14]

Proprioception and kinesthesia, the sensations that let you know the location of limbs while moving through space and that allow you to maintain your balance, are suggested to decline as one ages.[15] Relatedly, older adults exhibit greater postural sway and increased probability of losing balance and falling.[16] Thus, age-related decline in the kinesthetic receptors can occur.[17] Yet, falling may occur due to changes in central brain systems as well.[18] Falling is also associated with physical weakness, unsteady gait, mental confusion, and psychoactive drugs. While 40% of those 65 years and older living at home are reported to fall at least once each year, the rate steadily rises with age (about double for those 75 years and older), and is highest among those in long-term care institutions.[19] Basic fall prevention techniques include removing environmental tripping hazards, exercise, gait training, use of assistive walking devices, and discontinuation of medicines that cause orthostatic hypotension (i.e., low blood pressure when one stands up from sitting or lying down) or unnecessary sedation. Other more clinically directed preventions that focus on hypotension include sleeping with the head elevated, slowly rising, and sitting before standing as one gets out of bed, and use of orthopedic stockings to prevent venous pooling in the lower limbs.

As we encounter sensory-perceptual changes, we will need to adjust the activities and routines of our living. However, the inevitable changes and decline in sensory-perceptual processes need not mean that our celebration of life should be curtailed, nor savored less. Neither should our creative experiences and art-making be lessened or diminished as meaningful symbolisms of our living. Quite the contrary, despite the sensory-perceptual changes encountered, one may still live vibrantly, be more aware of one's freedom to act in accordance with one's own values, to create, and to drink in the richness of all life's moments.

Other Physical Changes and Risk for Disease

As we age our muscles decrease in strength, endurance, size, and weight relative to total body weight.[20] This change in physical capacity may impact upon one's creativity in several ways and may require us to find techniques that will help us maintain and strengthen muscles, as well as explore other avenues for creative expression. For example, singers may find that their range and ability to sing may change as vocal cords stiffen and vibrate at a higher frequency. For many of us in later life, the sound of our voices may be slightly higher and quaver due to loss of control over the vocal cords. In general, throughout the body, organ systems decline, and muscle fibers become stiffer and less resilient to healing due to the loss of collagen and molecular cross-linking. Eventually muscle is replaced with fat. Reflexes and reaction times slow due to both a decline in cognitive processes and in peripheral muscular-skeletal mechanics. Heart and lung function also decrease, dispensing oxygenated blood more slowly with advancing age.

Older adults who have physical disabilities, are very ill, who have cognitive or psychological disorders, and who need assistance in activities of daily living are generally defined as frail.[21] Indices of functionality include the Activities of Daily Living (ADL), a measure of basic self-care (e.g., eating, bathing, toileting, walking, dressing), and the Instrumental Activities of Daily Living (IADL), a measure that reflects our ability to live independently and which entails intellectual competence and executive planning (e.g., shopping for food, paying bills, making appointments, taking medications, going to the doctor).[22] As the older person encounters illness and changes in physical capacity, there is an increasing likelihood of functional limitations as defined by the ADL and IADL measures, and thus an increasing need for assistance. Factors such as a history of smoking, heavy drinking, physical inactivity, depression, social isolation, and poor health are all predictors that the person will likely become frail and require assistance.[23]

The types of medical problems we may encounter in later life also become of greater concern. As reported by the U.S. Centers for Disease Control and Prevention in 2021, the leading causes of death in the U.S. for individuals 65 years or older listed in prevalence were heart disease, cancers, Covid-19, cerebral vascular disease, Alzheimer's disease, and chronic respiratory diseases.[24] Moreover, many of us in later life will live with a variety of chronic conditions. Indeed, the U.S. National Council on Aging reported in 2021, that 80% of adults 65 years and older have one of the following common and most prevalent chronic conditions, and 68% of those over the age of 65 have two or more! These chronic conditions include arthritis, hypertensive disease, high cholesterol, hypertension, ischemic/coronary disease, diabetes, chronic kidney disease, heart failure, depression, Alzheimer's disease and dementia, and chronic obstructive pulmonary disease.[25]

Prevention behaviors that may allow us to avoid illness and extend our longevity include not smoking, eating a nutritious and balanced diet, getting enough sleep, exercising regularly, practicing safe-sex and other good safety habits (e.g., using seatbelts), partaking of alcohol in moderation, getting regular health check-ups, and avoiding sun and cold exposure. If we do these in conjunction with holding an optimistic outlook on life, staying involved with and maintaining social contacts, and continue to be active in our work and play, then we are also more likely to live rather happily and longer![26] Nevertheless, we must note that there are some concerns that are not easy to escape. For example, in developed countries like Australia, Canada, Germany, France, Norway, U.K., U.S.A., aging is implicated in the prevalent diseases of later life (i.e., heart disease, cancers, and neurodegenerative illnesses).[27] Further, access to health-care and medicines, as well as the socio-environmental context that surrounds us, also are noted to influence our health and longevity.[28] In low-income countries, communicable illnesses like diarrheal diseases, tuberculosis, and malaria are noted to rank high on the list for leading causes of death.[29] Thus, living in a community where medical care is available and medicines affordable, and where environmental conditions allow for a high quality of life and intellectual and creative engagement is important to our health and well-being, and in extending our longevity.

As we take up the question of what later life will bring, it is important to note that lifestyle affects risk for disease as well as immune function. Immunological research has indicated that the number of T-lymphocytes stays the same across the life span, however, as we age and these cells mature, they may be less able to "learn" to fight new invaders.[30] This is one reason why older are more prone to illness and disease than younger adults. Indeed, older adults take longer to produce cells that fight off viruses and build up an immunity against specific diseases, even after immunization. Further, stress and depression have been shown to change and exacerbate immune system functioning, making one more susceptible to illness and disease.[31] This is of particular concern for caregiving spouses and partners, who were found to have an increased risk for stroke and illness as they endured the stress of taking care of a partner with Alzheimer's disease.[32] Thus, we should be aware that chronic exposure to stressors negatively affect immune function.[33] Likewise, if we only view getting older in negative and deleterious ways, then our psychological construction of "aging" by itself may adversely affect and thus inhibit our immune functioning.[34]

Overcoming the Antagonist

We earlier noted a model of later life which characteristically depicts older people as medical patients, in a downward spiral of dependency, relying on the assistance of caregivers and family. Indeed, as Cicero also wrote many years ago, older adults are commonly portrayed in stereotypical ways and socially shunned, and these ageist expressions negatively impact the health of older adults.[35] Embracing the whole person approach, however, we recognize that self and identity are much more than the sum of all the facets that make up these constructs. From this orientation we may view our "selves" and others in a way that recognizes our adaptive nature, enduring characteristics, and life experiences, that in combination direct our feeling, thinking, and acting. We become aware of the infinite possibilities that yet exist for each of us as our lives unfold. Indeed, health challenges that occur in later life may force us to transition to different ways of living but also reveal novel aspects of oneself. For example, as we found in the story of Father Champlin in the last chapter, illness experiences may inspire a greater empathy and deeper spiritual faith, and stir within the person a broader sense of social belonging and appreciation of the many small yet good things in life.[36]

Thus, in contrast to models that centrally focus on the declines or deteriorations that may occur in later life, those that emphasize the whole person have put forth a more positive and resilient characterization of aging.[37] Underscoring, as many older adults often report, that there is much life and living to do beyond age 65.[38] Indeed, in older age we continue to strive for freedom and personal autonomy, expressing our own unique inner standards and personal beliefs. We still desire to execute our free will and direct our own living. We continue to need and nurture warm and satisfying relations with others, and to find significant meaning and purpose in our living. Further, perhaps understood in a different way later in life, we may seek deeper insight into and fulfillment through our moral beliefs and actions, as well as spiritual expressions.[39]

We propose that participation in creative activities can illuminate ways we may find new meaning and purpose in later life, and buffer us from the many sources of life stress. Further, our immersion in the arts may enrich and protectively extend our lives.[40] For example, research exploring the effect of art-making on induced stress reported significantly greater reduction in stress levels for subjects who were involved in artistic tasks.[41] Another study suggested that taking an acting class relieves stress and improves quality of life.[42] In research examining the effects of taking a 30-minute dance class, three times a week, for eight-weeks, participants reported significant decline in baseline measures of stress at the end of eight-weeks.[43] Similarly, other investigations have suggested art-making to induce a "creative high,"[44] and to buffer the existential stress associated with death anxiety.[45] Thus, through involvement with the arts we may discover our own and other's creativity, address existential concerns, and look toward a more positive future. In the next sections we share the stories of Rick Belcher, Meryl Shechter, Mitch Wadley, and Jim Weatherhead that highlight how music making may enrich our lives.

Blind Courage

It is not often we learn about what it is like to grow older and to be blind. Rick Belcher and Meryl Shechter, both amateur musicians, 69 years of age at the time of our meeting, and both blind since birth, were asked and agreed to share their story for this book.[46]

Rick Belcher is an outgoing, bold, and gregarious person, expressing a heroic manner as he often spoke of standing up for and defending others. He grew up listening to rhythm and blues on the black radio stations, and thus in many ways is a musical historian of that genre. He is also a self-taught pianist and rock and roll singer. He lived with his parents and siblings in Arkansas, until he was almost 40 years old, later moving to St. Louis, Missouri.

Meryl Shechter is a very talented, dynamic, and gracious person. She grew up in Long Island, New York, and like Rick has long been active in making music. Meryl took piano lessons for 12 years, first learning to play by ear. Later she studied French, Spanish, and music at Adelphi University. She learned to read music by using the Braille technique. Before retiring, Meryl worked for the U.S. Social Security Administration and the U.S. Internal Revenue Service, and at the time of our interview served as Vice President of the American Council of the Blind of Maryland.

As Rick and Meryl related in a series of conversations, being blind presents many challenges in life. However, they both noted that despite their disability, they are proud to be members of the blind community. During our discussions it was clear to recognize the bond of friendship they shared, and the deep concern and love they have for one another. Both had been in marriages before— Rick's first wife had passed away in 1999, and Meryl's earlier marriage had ended in divorce. They both related how these were very difficult and emotionally challenging episodes for them, and would occasionally surface during our conversations. Rick would speak of his great love for Maui, his late wife. Meryl would allude to the hurt and marital strife she experienced. So, in many ways their friendship was calling them both into new ways of being in later life. They share many interests, and one of their great joys is music, especially playing and singing together. They first met each other briefly when they visited the World Services for the Blind in Little Rock, Arkansas. But in 2018, they both attended an American Council of the Blind meeting in St. Louis and started dating. Later, they became engaged.

As a musician, since the 1990s Rick has played piano and sang at jazz bars and in nursing homes in the St. Louis area, and with Meryl they performed as a duo for the *Evening of Entertainment* produced by the St. Louis Recreational Council for Disabilities in 2018. One special radio performance was in August 2021, when Meryl sang a French folk song, and Rick played keyboard and sang a rock ballad on the American Council of the Blind's *ACB Radio*

Media 5 station, an interactive radio program for the blind. As they related to the interviewer, music brought them together. Discussing their music making, Rick noted, "I love to perform and play the blues, and when I perform, I want people to enjoy themselves. You have to feel the blues to be able to sing the blues." Meryl added that "Rick is in a trance when he performs—heart and soul, and he doesn't think about anything else." For both Rick and Meryl music is a central facet of their identity. The repertoire of songs performed by Rick are those that address personal freedoms and take on social issues and sing of overcoming. Meryl also noted that for her, "Music is a way to express my Jewishness," and added, some of her favorite songs are songs that express concern for social justice and include Bob Dylan's "Blowing in the Wind" as well as the folk music of Pete Seeger, Woodie Guthrie, Steve Paxton, and Joni Mitchell.

Throughout our discussions both Rick and Meryl expressed a deep interpersonal sensitivity, and a great vitality and joy in living. Always with great enthusiasm, they shared an outlook on life that seemed ageless. In our conversation they conveyed how other sensory modalities were more accentuated in how they perceived the world. For example, Meryl related that in her mind's eye she could feel and sense what it would be like to hold and taste a cheeseburger. They also enjoyed sharing their understandings of life, as Rick termed it, "sharing insights without sight." Asked what they found stressful in later life, both Rick and Meryl noted access to transportation and getting around town was one of their biggest aggravations. Regarding how these issues affected everyday living, Rick noted, "all the hassles like going to the bank, doing laundry, etc., that a normal person may confront, are ten-times harder for someone with a disability."

Reflecting on what they learned in life so far, Rick said "to be your own person—explore the world. Life is what you make it. Be happy where you are and love your family." Meryl added, "Life throws you lots of curve balls… and life teaches you—both your head and your heart… and while there are ups and downs, when you are down you can always get up again!" As we continued to talk, our discussions shifted more to listening to songs that Rick and

Meryl would sing. As they both approached the seventh decade of their lives, each expressed a strong sense of self-autonomy, and a great desire to continue to live independently and to explore the world. They also expressed an excitement about their next adventures in life, opportunities to be creative, and, at the age of 69, the exhilaration of being engaged to one another and what may occur in the future. Rick told us that he had purchased a ring and proposed to Meryl as he visited her at Thanksgiving time. They talked of the future which included planning vacations and looking forward to the joys of living together. Undefeated by blindness Rick and Meryl are courageously taking on the challenges of later life, as they express how music and the love they share for one another has brought them deep fulfillment and joy.

In further talks with Rick and Meryl they also discussed the many special navigational procedures required for those who are blind. Using a walking stick, Meryl related how she would practice walking to the bus stop to learn the route, so that she could then use the bus to take her to work. She noted the high degree of orienting needed to learn the many steps to the bus stop, the places where she would cross different streets and boulevards safely, and the point at which the bus would stop for her to board. It was an orienting activity that had to be learned and rehearsed. Rick mentioned times when he had been a victim of muggers and almost run over when crossing the street. He also noted that, occasionally, when some sighted strangers offered help, it was more challenging than just being left alone. Rick also instructed that the best practice for giving assistance to a blind person is to offer your arm for them to use as a following guide. Then, as you may also do with anyone who is visually impaired, announce upcoming steps, doorways, or other changes in the path or environment that will need to be navigated. Avoid guiding by pushing or pulling. As Rick related, much like a dance, "You can lead and I will follow, but if you start directing me by use of physical force, pushing and pulling, then it is more likely that you are treating me much like a plow. Please don't do that!" Again, the best practice is to offer your arm to grasp and use as a following guide.

Other disabilities such as hearing loss negatively affect physical and emotional well-being, and social functioning.[47] As we become aware of a person's hearing impairment, we may consider the following ways to help: Encourage use of assisted hearing devices that allow amplification of sound levels, such as headsets that are available at museums, theatres, and concert halls. During conversation, find a quiet place to talk, and clearly articulate the sounds of your speech, but not in a deliberately slowed or affected manner. Let the person see your face so they can read your lips and use facial cue information to aid them in understanding your communication. Speak in the lower-register of your voice-range to reduce problems the other person may have in picking up high-pitched speech sounds and be patient and repeat yourself if necessary. Be careful to project your voice, but don't shout or yell. As many may have experienced, being yelled at is psychologically assaulting and does not convey our positive regard for the person.

Other types of accommodations, such as encouraging use of and providing access to hearing aids has been suggested to reduce symptoms of depression and improve quality of life for those with hearing impairment.[48] Similarly, recommending use of magnifying glasses, telescoping spectacles, video magnifiers, as well as non-optical conversion of everyday tools so that they are "bigger-bolder-brighter" (e.g., use of large print books, high contrast watches, reading stands) is another way of accommodating. These types of accommodations aid individuals with low vision and can enhance quality of life.[49] Further, behavioral and psychosocial accommodations like those described above are also noted to assist vision and hearing impaired individuals in coping and making positive adjustment to declines in sensory functioning.[50] Further, these accommodations can also benefit caregivers as they provide assistance.

* * *

Plot-Twists and Finding New Creative Pathways

This is the Professor speaking—coming to you directly from the other-side of the wilderness... Now who wants to know what Red has in her basket?" - Professor Mitch Wadley, from "Little Red Riding Hood (Featuring the Paper Bag) [51]

On a warm July day, in the late-1990s, a drummer and bass-player sang and played funky music on the sidewalk along Delmar Boulevard in St. Louis, Missouri. Singing a unique and mirth-filled song, the bass-player intoned about "Little Red Riding Hood" and something she had in her basket. Was it a chitlin sandwich? Or, as the song suggested, something else? The funky song was a new take on the classic childhood story about Little Red Riding Hood and the Big Bad Wolf. While appreciating their avant-garde style of dress and theatrical performance, one may not have thought much more about these street buskers, except that one of the author's fiancé at the time, and now wife, mentioned that the drummer was the daughter of her godfather and family friend! So, naturally there was more to know about the performers and their music. Thus, that first encounter started a series of meetings and conversations that, in preparation for this book, culminated in a more formal interview with Professor Mitch Wadley, the bass-player.[52]

Professor Mitch Wadley's story, like many of the life stories the reader knows, involves a long journey, the encountering of great challenges, redirections along the way and new paths to follow, with enduring hopes of finding success and coming to a happy ending. Using the title of "Professor" as his performing appellation, and not as an academic designation, in a conversation about his music and career, we learn more about Professor Mitch Wadley's story.

Professor Mitch Wadley's Story

Born in 1951, Professor Mitch Wadley is a talented older musician, who grew up listening to the rhythm and blues bands in St. Louis, Missouri, and later jammed and played with the likes of Jimi Hendrix, Buddy Cox, and B.B. King in New York City at the end of the 1960s. Early in his life, as Mitch was expanding his artistic palette, he turned his ear toward the very distinctive musical expressions of soul and funk music. Developing a mastery of the electric bass, and composing and singing his own songs, by his early 20s Mitch was a member of The 13th Floor, a soul and funk band from St. Louis. The band included a unique collection of musical geniuses, recruited by Oliver Sain Jr. as the back-up band for the Blues and Rock Hall of Fame guitarist Albert King, as he prepared for a concert tour in the Northeast U.S. in the mid-1970s. The funky disco sound and resultant musical acclaim of The 13th Floor soon had them opening for top acts like Funkadelic, Curtis Mayfield, the Staple Sisters, and the group WAR. In 1977, the band released their only album, entitled *Steppin' Out* on the Blue Candle label. Recognized as part of the classic-funk and groove genre since 2012, and often selling-out all copies of their compact disc and vinyl record pressings, The 13th Floor's *Steppin' Out* has been reissued as a compact disc in Japan three times, and on vinyl in the United Kingdom once. On the album, Mitch is sole author of the song "Teffany," and shares authorship on "Hang Loose," "Steppin' Out," "Leanin'," and "Gina lako nani." However, "making it" in the music industry can be difficult, and while many artists may hold rights to the songs they write, they may not always own the rights to or receive royalties from the music they recorded. This was the case for members of The 13th Floor, and thus despite the group's initial success in making a record, the band soon disbanded and its members pursued other interests.

For Mitch there were also serious health challenges on the horizon. In his early 30s he was diagnosed with and underwent successful neurosurgery for a benign brain tumor. As noted earlier, health problems often constitute an existential crisis for the person, and indeed this was the case for Mitch. Illness diagnoses, surgeries, and recovery processes can all be life-altering events, taking precedent over and redirecting one's everyday activities, and as in Mitch's case, represents a significant plot-twist in his story. Nevertheless, after successful surgery and with health restored, Mitch continued his musical career, and in the mid-1980s composed and recorded a collection of funk, blues, gospel, and country songs that included, "Broke All the Time," "God's Victory," "A Love

Called Mine," "Singin' Down the Road," "Joey," "Little Red Riding Hood," "May the Whole World Dance," "Ooh, Ooh, 'Baby I Love Ya'," and "Professor's Funk." Always in love with music, and with the assistance of friends in the recording industry, Mitch produced a re-recording of his songs with the intention of "re-claiming" rights to all his music. This new recording was released in 2019 as the digital MP3 album *Extra Terrestrial Fonk* on TuneCore, a digital platform that helps musical artists independently distribute, publish, and license their music.[53] Describing this new album, Professor Mitch refers to it as "my masterpiece," and, after many years of sacrifice and dedication, the songs that appear on the CD and MP3 album are an incredible artistic accomplishment! As music lovers throughout the world have expressed, Professor Mitch's songs tell a story that speaks to our current moment. Indeed, they acknowledge the many challenges of our modern living, and yet express an extraordinarily rich celebration of life and the joy that we may find in listening to and making music together.

In our conversations about his musical career, Mitch noted that as he enters his seventh decade of life he no longer has the ability to play or perform like he once did. Yet, he is still interested in helping others make and produce music—and he still has the creative savvy to make very funky music! However, due to physical changes, the instrument he was currently playing and exploring at the time of our interview was the bongo drum. As Mitch talked, he expressed an understanding of life gained through all the health and artistic challenges he encountered. He expressed a strong religious faith and deep gratitude for having recovered from his earlier health crisis, for each day of life, and for having good friends. Further, he spoke with excitement as he described producing and re-recording his music, and in making it available through various digital platforms. He voiced a hope that people would yet discover and be inspired by his music, and that perhaps other musicians might choose a song or two to record on their next albums. As we talked Mitch proclaimed that what inspires his life now, and as he also describes in his aptly named song, is the miracle of "God's Victory." Still singing as he moves down life's road, Mitch happily expressed, "my life is in God's hands," and shared an enthusiasm for "seeing what comes next." In talking with Professor Mitch, a sense of accepting life on its own terms is conveyed. Mitch's story reminds us of the plot-twists we may encounter as we face health challenges and find ourselves on new paths to travel. Many of us will do battle with the antagonists of physical decline and illness—the ones that stalk us and intrude into our deepest thoughts, seeking to upset our rational orientation of acceptance and feelings about how we might live, and how we might relate to the world and become in later life. Yet, as we encounter challenges such as these, we may also find solace in knowing that we are adaptive beings, led to discover new insights. So as Professor Mitch's song teases at the beginning of this section, what *is* in Little Red Riding Hood's basket? We will reason about this at the end of the chapter, but first let us consider another story of plot-twists and life-redirections, and battle against the monster of illness.

Jim Weatherhead and His "Magic Carpet Ride"

We reported on and told many personal stories in our first book, *Music, Wellness, and Aging: Defining, Directing, and Celebrating Life.*[54] Each portrayed a person in development and in the process of becoming. Further, in many ways each account became a distinct tile that inlayed and intersected in a mosaic suggesting how people use the power of music in directing, defining, and celebrating their life. A similar story gathered for this book comes from Jim Weatherhead, a life-long fan of the rock group Steppenwolf and John Kay. In his own words, Jim relates his development, his living with chronic pain, and his magic carpet ride with music. It is a story of relationships and of hope, of plot-twists and new paths, of living with illness and overcoming pain, and of involvement with music throughout life:

> Like many that grew up in the late 60's early 70's, I had a great time as a pre-teen boy with the neighbor girls listening to "pop AM top 40" – which was my introduction to music, and girls! – a combination that sealed the deal on a lifelong music passion.

I recall my earliest musical dreams were of playing the trumpet. Herb Albert and the Tijuana Brass was a big thing in my childhood, the only music I ever heard mom say she liked. I used to sing and whistle the song "Winchester Cathedral" constantly, and even today that song will loop in my mind every so often. I had a "hipster aunt" that used to play records on our rare visits. I remember Booker T and the MG's "Green Onions" as being the first song to make me want to move and groove—thank you Aunt Minnie!

My mother was not a music fan, and it was just her and I living a very basic existence that didn't leave room for the arts nor the means for me to buy a trumpet and join the school band. I sang in choir at school but felt the peer pressure of "being cool" and regrettably quit. So dumb.

I had a friend that picked up a guitar and started playing along with Johnny Cash. I decided that I wanted to play the drums; I used to sneak into the band room at school and play the kettle drums and loved how the pitch could be changed, both by pedal and where the head was struck. I had to find a way to play music.

I sold greeting cards door to door; I only had to sell 25 boxes to get a drum kit! It was cold work in the early Minnesota winter and took what seemed like forever to sell 25 expensive boxes. I was so happy when I reached the goal and ordered the drum kit. It took a very long time for the drum kit to show up and when it did the disappointment was crushing — it was a tiny sized, super cheaply built kid kit. I should have known better. Regardless, I tried to play it and broke it almost instantly. I was simply too big physically and struck the heads far too hard. It was spring, and so my focus changed to bicycles and sports. Learning to play music would have to wait. As it turned out the wait was many decades.

I was about 12 and started to work and make my own money. I bought an RCA portable record player and went to the small-town drug store to buy my first "real" 33 rpm album. Paging through the very limited selection, I stumbled onto Steppenwolf's *At Your Birthday Party*... and I thought, that's the one for me! These guys look cool – the song titles also caught my youthful "rebel" eye...

Steppenwolf's "Rock Me" was the very song that moved music into my deeper soul. Music became my church. The song's lyrics introduced me to the depth that music has to enlighten and calm rage and anger that, for some, cannot be calmed in other healthy ways. Sadly, I did not return to the drums or any other instrument... Still music absorbed every pore as I came of age and lived my life. Music became my spiritual partner. I was a fan and consumer, but not a playing artist or musician.

I lived with folk musicians in my early 20's and lived the dream vicariously through them. Looking back, I'm surprised that for whatever reason, I didn't aspire to learn to play then or even sing, I was just content to be in the circle and serve as support "staff."

Ankylosing Spondylitis (AS) became my beast of burden. During my entire twenties and thirties, I was in constant and severe pain, and during the slow debilitating physical loss that consumed me, music was always there as a refuge for my tortured mind.

As I learned to live with pain, which I think is mostly a spiritual journey, I started to make adaptations to keep my passions alive. As a very physically orientated person this was difficult, and it seemed, at first, almost impossible to find a balance. Music was always there to help me relax, as an escape, or to jump start my energy and get me moving when I could barely walk or get out of bed.

I'm thankful that narcotic pain medication was not an option that was prescribed for chronic pain during my worst years – the mid-1980s through the late-1990s. I was able to use cannabis, combined with yoga (breath-work), and music, all kinds of music, to calm the chaos of a mind consumed by physical pain and spiritual demons.

My own musical journey did not start until much later in my life. I turned 50 and decided that if I was ever

115

going to become a musician, I could not wait another moment. I still wanted to play the drums but given the hip and shoulder issues I live with, decided that they may not be the best choice. I've always enjoyed piano and organ music and thought the traditional piano lesson path would be the way forward.

I started out taking lessons at ground zero. It was hard, very hard, and I struggled mightily to find smooth connection or flow between my mind's focus and the music on the sheet. I would get lost. I didn't "feel" any connection between the music in my mind and the chords on the keyboard, let alone the separation between the right and left hands. It took me a long, long time to "feel" the song beyond robotically playing the notes on paper. I started to get very frustrated. I'm generally very gifted when it comes to learning new skills – that was most certainly not the case with music. A lifetime of deep appreciation and a mind filled with song did not translate to learning the skills needed to be a musician.

I finally started to make a connection with some basic blues chords and a 12-bar structure that had me finally playing "real" songs, very simple songs, but it was my first feeling that I had made a step forward to believe that I could indeed play. It was not long after that I was writing the "Blessed Man's Journey," a story in which I used musical practice as a metaphor to describe the long hard journey to acceptance of living with pain and the resulting crippling effects of AS. Like a struggling musician that suddenly believes he can play, the long hours of struggle, practice and commitment do "pay off."

Ultimately, I was still frustrated. I started playing the harmonica to break up the frustrations – frustrations mostly centered on my lack of skill building on the keyboard. The harmonica allowed me to freelance, and "feel" music in a way I could not seem to reach on the keyboard. I took some voice lessons and started to sing.

116

As my body was feeling better now that the biologic medication became more and more effective, I decided that I'd have more fun playing the drums than continuing to "force" myself to play keyboards—I say force because it had started not to be fun. I needed to make a course correction.

I took to the drums pretty fast. Again, it took some time to bridge the feel of robotic play to actually feeling and fully occupying the beat and groove. I'm blessed with good "time" and have a lot of fun with the drums, even if I do still tend to flip the beat too often after a fill or beat transition. I love how I hear music now as I search for structure and nuance, music is such an amazing art form.[55]

Jim's story again makes us aware of the existential challenges of illness and the many ways our lives may become redirected. It also exemplifies how music may be a balm for the spirit as well as a therapeutic aid for dealing with pain. Further, as Jim's story implicitly suggests, we are never too old to try something new, even taking up a new musical instrument!

* * *

Jim Weatherhead also offers this reflective poem about music and his life:

Math Counts Music's Soul

Math counts music's soul
Skip in five, sharps right flats left
Keynote circles fifths

In life, his choice was
to drum. Had only to count
in fours – many ways

His seven-stroke roll
swung past the triplet bronze tones
and a waltz broke out

Sticks with pad must play
Paradiddle's rudiments
Rhythmic timing fun [56]

What Does Red Have in Her Basket?

In the classic story from childhood, *Little Red Riding Hood*, our protagonist Red is up against the Big Bad Wolf and seems unafraid as she visits her grandmother. In her narration of what is occurring, she expresses unabashed courage as she looks into the face of the monster. Metaphorically, as suggested by Professor Mitch Wadley in his song, Red holds something special in her basket. Symbolic of a deeper psychic reality, the song's lyrics leaves the listener thinking that, "that something," is our inherent qualities to be adaptive and creative, to hold hope and strive to overcome, and to attain the prize we seek. As expressed, both in its syncopated beat and harmonic structure, as well as in verse, Professor Mitch's song states, "Red has the funk!" Similarly, as told in the stories of Rick Belcher, Meryl Shechter, Mitch Wadley, and Jim Weatherhead, despite the curve balls we are thrown or the plot-twists that shift our life onto new pathways, the challenges of health crises and aging declines are not all-defeating or eclipsing of our powers of self-agency. Rather, they introduce and become connected with new insights and understandings as we struggle to overtake them. Indeed, these challenges may compel us to revise what we hold dear and what direction our lives will take. As Cicero alluded, they may also allow us to become aware of the advantages of getting older, and help us discover new areas of enjoyment and a deeper appreciation for living.

SEVEN — MOVE DOWNSTAGE LEFT — THEN WALK TO CENTER

All theatre actors learn that the way they walk and travel on the stage is designed to tell a story. With a pause in movement, or direction to the next stage mark, the actor communicates a message to the audience. Their movements reveal an emotion that is felt or makes a dramatic punctuation of the scene or plot. Indeed, there is an art to "walking." How we "walk" is also a metaphor for the way we hope to be in life. In this allegorical expression, each step shows where we have been, and points to where we may be headed. As we reflect upon our personal journey, we can recognize how far we have traveled, and the key milestones we have passed along the way. We may remember times when we felt we were racing ahead, or felt we were falling behind. At times we may have been unsure where we were going, and had to find our balance again to move on in a positive way. We may also recollect times when we were able to linger for a while, were inspired, and felt a special significance about our experience. Walking is indeed a metaphor for our life. It is through this "art of walking" that we link mind, body, and spirit, achieve balance in all we do, and find a deeper understanding of who we are.

The Art of Walking

Henry David Thoreau in his essay *Walking*, praises the great pastoral beauty and restorative effect found in Nature as he travels through its forested cathedrals and across its hallowed prairies and plains. Indeed, he writes, "There is a subtle magnetism in Nature, which, if we unconsciously yield to it, will direct us aright."[1] Nature's majestic mountains, awe-inspiring oceans, and waters of rebirth remind us of our mutual dependence and connection with the natural world. As Thoreau further noted, in our walks and contact with the great outdoors we may discover many things to appreciate and marvel in. We may find wonder in the inordinate beauty of birdsong melodies, or the pleasure of watching frolicking faunae. We may be amazed by the lightning bolt as it travels across the sky or its resultant thunderclap. We may sense a tranquility in the calmness of a light breeze, or feel awe as we witness the power of a gale.

In our walk and encounter with Nature, we may experience physical invigoration as well as a relaxation and easiness that allows healing to arise from the depths of our unconscious mind. Thus, walking is recognized as a method of maintaining and enhancing our physical health as well as psychological and emotional well-being. As Thoreau celebrated, we need to spend time outdoors, to find and discover a oneness that we share with Nature, so that we can move beyond the demands and stressors of our worldly engagements and enterprises. When we recognize our connection with Nature, we become attuned to the temperament of the seasons, and sense the vastness of time that guides stars and planets. As many nature walkers have described, our experiences in the great outdoors reveal to us a sacredness about life, ourselves, and the world that surrounds us. A sacredness, Thoreau noted, that shines a light into our minds and hearts that is as warm, serene, and brilliant as the sunshine on an Autumn Day.

Biophysical and Other Benefits of Walking

More often discussed as a technical method than an art, walking and other physical exercises are recommended as both a prevention and management routine for a wide range of illness and disease.[2] Thus, walking is noted as an essential practice of a healthy lifestyle. For example, an investigation of mobility and balance in older adults found that at 75 years of age, walking-gait speed predicted 10-year survival for both older men and women.[3] Furthermore, this same investigation suggested walking speed to be as important a predictor of mortality risk as is age, chronic health conditions, use of mobility aids, and other predictive factors such as history of tobacco use, blood pressure, body mass index, and history of hospitalization. In addition, slower walking speed was also found to predict greater postoperative morbidity and one-year mortality in patients following cardiac and colorectal surgeries.[4] However, a leisurely strolling type of walking may not be sufficient to realize all the protective advantages of this type of exercise. For example, one study has suggested that for older men it may be necessary to either walk for an hour a day or at a faster pace (at or above 3.2 km/h, or 2 mph) to reap all the physical benefits of walking.[5] Thus, as a basic exercise, brisk walking is distinguished as the physical-core exercise prescriptive in managing hypertension, heart disease, diabetes, and other chronic illnesses.[6]

Further, walking is also noted to aid mental functioning and psychological well-being. For example, in a U.S. sample of 1,700 adults 65 years of age or older, getting regular exercise by walking, hiking, cycling, or other aerobic activities three or more times a week was associated with decreased risk for dementia, with the greatest risk reduction found in individuals at low physical performance levels.[7] Allied research that examined the benefits of walking in a sample of Japanese American men 71 to 93 years of age, also indicated a reduction in risk for dementia; this reduction was noted in groups that walked more than 2 miles a day, or as little as .25 to 1 mile a day.[8] Further, in a randomized control trial of older adults in Japan, where participants were encouraged to walk on a regular basis over the course of three months, in comparison to control subjects who did not walk regularly, members of the walking group demonstrated better word fluency, functional capacity, social interaction, and motor function.[9] Leading the researchers to suggest that walking may enhance some aspects of cognition, functional capacity, and quality-of-life, and thus may be a useful intervention to maintain one's vitality and prevent or slow mental decline.

Walking often takes us into the great outdoors, which may provide its own unique benefits. For example, in reviews of the literature that compared the psychological effects of exercising indoors versus outdoors, exercising in natural environments has been found to be associated with increased energy and greater feelings of revitalization and positive engagement, and decreases in negative affective states such as anger and sadness.[10] Walking is also a simple exercise that we can do alone or with others, so it may respectively provide both a time when we can be alone to reflect deeply on issues of concern as well as an opportunity for social exchange and supportive social interactions. Moreover, when we consider walking and social companionship, it is worth noting that for pet-owners, even the task of walking the dog is suggested to provide a regularity of exercise that is beneficial to personal health.[11]

Treks: Great and Small

What are other ways we can engage in the art of walking? A great trek such as hiking the Appalachian Trail, an approximately 2,190-mile (3,525 km) route that runs continuously from its northernmost point of Mount Katahdin in Maine to its southernmost point of Springer Mountain in Georgia, is one example of how we might participate in the art of walking. As noted in many books about hiking the Appalachian Trail, not only does one encounter the wilds of nature and gain first-hand knowledge of the fauna, flora and geographic features of the Eastern United States, but also one may rediscover a sense of one's true self.[12] Indeed, many thru-hikers, those individuals who walked the entire length of the trail, often report their motivation for walking was to test one's self against the "roughing-it" demands of the trail, to learn about and to know oneself better, to grow as a person, to make a life transition to greater understanding, and to encounter and realize a spiritual experience.[13] Further, this experience is one that has involved many older adults. For example, of the over 21,500 thru-hikers of the Appalachian Trail since the first one in 1936, 750 were in their 60s. Fifty individuals were in their 70s, and 2 hikers in their 80s with the oldest being 82 years of age. The first female solo thru-hiker was Emma Gatewood, better known to fellow trail hikers as "Grandma Gatewood," mother of 11 children and 23 grandchildren, who at the age of 67 first hiked the trail in 1955. Grandma Gatewood later thru-hiked the trail at age 69 in 1957, and in 1964 completed the trail a third time by doing smaller treks, or sectional hikes, at the age of 75.[14] Undoubtedly, to hike from one end of the Appalachian Trail to the other represents a walk of a lifetime, and perhaps one of the greatest personal accomplishments imaginable at any age!

Sail Away

As Nicola Rodriguez's instructs in her book *Sail Away: How to Escape the Rat Race and Live the Dream*, sailing is another activity that allows us to encounter the many wonders of nature and to find an insight into ourselves.[15] Sailing is perhaps the most ancient of methods, and farthest-reaching of the great treks. Historically, we recognize Homer's account of the grand journey undertaken by Odysseus, King of Ithaca, where unknown challenges of the sea lay bare the archetypes of mind, exposing a deeper way of knowing and understanding ourselves. Indeed, in many sea-faring tales we learn about the mysteries of the deep, the many perils of the journey that lay before the sojourner, coupled with temptations and torment of mind and flesh, characteristic identifications of monsters and villains, and the courage of heroes and rescuers that point a way beyond ourselves, to a transcendent and eternal truth that will return us to a point of equilibrium and calm again. In more contemporary times, we hear of both extended as well as short sailing journeys, purposefully conducted to discover and know better the universe within oneself.[16]

Like hiking, those who sail include a wide range of individuals from many diverse backgrounds. As reported by the U.S. Sailing Organization, 56% of its members are 50 years of age or older.[17] Further, similar to Grandma Gatewood's great treks on the Appalachian Trail, older adults are also recognized for their long-distance sailing. For example, as recently as 2016, Bill Meanly of San Diego, California, at age 70 completed the Transpacific Yacht Race—where he single-handedly sailed from San Pedro, California, to Diamond Head in Hawaii, 2,225 nautical miles (2,560 land miles; or, 4,121 kilometers).[18] Thus, age alone is not necessarily a limiting factor for sailing. One person that has helped to redefine the boundaries of what is possible in later life is Jim Boren of Marinette, Wisconsin. In 2015, Jim at the age of 90-years old procured a 30-foot sailboat he christened *Skoal,* and single-handedly sailed his boat throughout the year on various cruises and races in the Great Lakes region of the United States.[19]

While not everyone has the time, strength, stamina, or motivation to hike or to sail such great distances. Hiking just a section of a favorite trail at a time, or making short trips from one port to another, may be more practical and more feasible later in life. Indeed, the short-distance sectional hikers of the Appalachian trail tend to be those who are older, with the median age being around 40 years. Furthermore, a variety of individuals with disabilities, and sojourners who were blind, with amputations above the knee, with diabetes, and recipients of organ transplants have completed the Appalachian Trail. Thus, age nor disability need stand in the way of individuals who seek this type of experience.

Similarly, short cruises across lakes or along shorelines are nearby and in reach of many sailors. Especially for older sailors, the catamaran (a bi-hull sailing vessel) offers accessibility and stability and has a shallow draft that allows it to sail close to beautiful shorelines and delightful lagoons.[20] Thus, sailing for older adults, either solo or as a member of a crew, may also be an encounter with nature that is both invigorating and transformative as the long-distance treks.

In our communion with nature and through the experiences of hiking or sailing, we may measure ourselves relative to the majesty of the steepest mountains, the widest oceans and deepest seas, the seemingly endless plains, and the infinite expanse of the sky. As a result, we recognize our smallness in the universe and are compelled to look inward to realize a deeper sense of being. In a short walk, or on longer hikes and sailing expeditions, we may discover unique opportunities to grow in knowledge of ourselves and the world we share with others. Other regimens that emphasize the art of movement such as the Chinese practices of tai chi and qigong, also recognize how physical activity may enhance our health and well-being, and we take those up next.

Tai Chi and Qigong

Tai chi, also known as taiji or taijiquan, and qigong are ancient Chinese physical exercise systems designed to integrate one's mind, body, and spirit. Their practice is traced as far back as 5000 BCE. The literal translation refers to a method of accessing "qi" (pronounced "chee"), a great and ultimate energy. Considered a basic exercise, a martial art, and a spiritual practice, tai chi and qigong emphasize detailed choreographed and flowing meditative movements that are coupled with rhythmic breathing to build physical strength and stamina, to achieve an inner balance, and to develop a sense of harmony with the natural and supernatural worlds. Drawing upon thousands of movements and routines (or forms), tai chi and qigong exercises may include actions and postures that mimic the movement and poses of animals, or the shadow boxing and defensive stances of martial arts, as well as the use of military weapons such as the crossbow, spear, or saber. The beneficial physiological, psychological, and spiritual effects of tai chi and qigong are suggested to be realized through an increase in fortitude and endurance, and finding a balance between positive and negative forces represented within nature. Thus, just as Thoreau alludes that nature's subtle magnetism may beneficially direct us in a way of being, the practices of tai chi and qigong similarly propose that as we act in sympathy with universal forces and rhythms, we may realize a harmony that enhances our mental and emotional well-being and directs us in our way of living.

To gain insight into these ancient practices and their personal benefit, we interviewed Professor Robert G. Santee, a counseling psychologist and scholar in Asian philosophy, as well as practitioner and teacher of tai chi and qigong. Discussing how he began to learn about tai chi and qigong practices, he also shares his personal observations and benefits of these exercises.

Robert G. Santee's Story

I entered the University of Hawaii (UH) in the Fall of 1970. At UH we had a one-credit physical education requirement for graduation, and on the recommendation of a friend, I took a one-credit class from a teacher named T. Y. Pang on the traditional Yang style of tai chi. After the completion of the course, I attended his off-campus class for a little over a year. His class was an eye-opener, and he was quite dynamic. In Honolulu, early on in 1978, I received private instruction in the traditional Wu (a method involving short physical sparring movements and the development of soft

126

internal energy) and Yang (a method involving larger physical sparring movements and the development of half hard and half soft internal energy) styles of tai chi, including the use of traditional straight and broad swords, and zhan zhuang qigong (a standing meditation with breathing control) from a tai chi teacher named T. C. Lee.

In 2004, I started taking classes from Zhijian Sifu Cai from Fujian, China, who was teaching classes in the new standardized forms of tai chi from China. In Honolulu, I also began taking classes in baguazhang (a martial art style that incorporates specific stepping, postures, and hand movements for fighting) from Laoshi (teacher) Zhang Xiu from Beijing, China. I attended with her and classmates, training with experts and masters that she had set up in Beijing, China, in 2007, 2009, and 2011. Over the course of this training in Beijing, I learned and studied the Cheng style baguazhang (a style of martial arts that incorporates different hand positions such as the claw and dragon), Yin style baguazhang (the art of striking while moving), sitting baduanjin qigong (a collection of sitting postures and movements to build strength, open energy channels, and improve health), standardized sun style tai chi (a martial art style with smooth flowing movements that omits vigorous jumping or crouching), standing baduanjin qigong (standing postures to enhance health, build strength, and optimize energy), standardized 42 form tai chi (a collection of physical movements and poses), and tai chi yangsheng staff qigong (movements with a staff). Over the years, Sifu Cai gradually had me assist him in teaching. Upon his recommendation in 2011, I was certified in the province of Fujian, China, a Wushu Jiaolian (trainer/coach). I am currently a senior instructor in the Xiaxing Martial Arts Association of Honolulu.

I have been consistently practicing tai chi and qigong for 17 years. Personal benefits for me consist of increased physical and psychological health and well-being, reduction in negative self-talk and mind wandering, increased flexibility, stress reduction and prevention, and increased focus, attention, and concentration. Other benefits include a freeing and opening of my mind, being more in harmony, and having a sense of peace and an embodied understanding. Most of these benefits I teach as being more deeply integrated with an ever-changing, interdependent, impermanent, and essentially empty process, that I flow through and that I simply hold an awareness of, as flowing through the present.

While I cannot speak for others, the literature seems to suggest that for those who are committed and dedicated to these practices on a consistent basis, the expressive bodily movements of tai chi and qigong are ways to direct and define one's lifestyle. In fact, the practice of tai chi and qigong does not stop with simply performing the various forms and postures. It becomes integral to everything you do during your daily life. There is no question that the more you correctly practice on a consistent basis, over time, the forms, and postures themselves open up to you an endless process of discovery and awe. [21]

Biophysical, Neurocognitive, and Psychological Effects

Of note are physical changes that may occur through tai chi and qigong practices (e.g., a general strengthening of muscle and enhanced stamina, strengthening of muscles that are used in preventing falling, increase in bone density) that lead to greater mobility and independence in later life, as well as positive neurobiological effects.[22] For example, randomized control trial research examining the effects of tai chi training on balance reported an improvement in walking gait suggested to help mitigate fall risk in healthy older adults.[23] Further, other research involving older adults with chronic illness who practiced qigong exercises in a group, reported reduction in depressive symptoms while also noting enhanced grip strength and self-report of physical well-being.[24] Additionally, two meta-reviews (i.e., a systematic review of many different studies) involving normal healthy older adults and those with cognitive impairment reported that tai chi exercise may significantly improve various aspects of cognition such as memory and learning, speed of processing and attention, mental flexibility, and visuospatial perception of older adults with cognitive impairment.[25] Thus, tai chi exercises are suggested to offer cognitive benefits for both healthy and cognitively impaired older adults.

During warm weather, it is often common to see older adults in city parks practicing tai chi and qigong in groups. Considering different effects of these exercises when performed in a group or alone, Professor Santee offers:

> Given that we are wired via the process of evolution to belong to groups, as group membership enhances our chances of survival, of finding a mate, reproducing, passing on our gene pool and maintaining it, I suspect there are significant neurotransmitter and hormonal changes that occur providing positive reinforcement so that we continue to engage in belonging to groups. So, doing tai chi and/or qigong in a group clearly can, independent of the tai chi or qigong, have a positive effect on you.
>
> In addition to the positivity of group membership, tai chi and qigong are often practiced outside in nature. Being in nature has a clear positive impact, in most cases, on how we feel physically and psychologically. Clearly this is also part of our evolutionary wiring, and I suspect there are significant neurotransmitter and hormonal changes that occur providing positive reinforcement. I have presented papers on Daoism at conferences in Hong Kong, as well as in the cities of Tiantai, Chengdu, Wudang, and Changsha in China, and in Taiwan on Cross Cultural Counseling, and visited major cities in China such as Beijing, Shanghai, and Hangzhou. Invariably, in the early morning, I would see hundreds of people in the parks, mostly elderly, in large and small groups, and some alone, practicing primarily tai chi and qigong. In 2020, tai chi was inscribed by UNESCO (United Nations Educational, Scientific and Cultural Organization) on the representative list of the intangible

cultural heritage of humanity. Tai chi has had considerable impact throughout the world with an estimated 400 million practitioners. In my opinion, most people who practice tai chi and qigong consistently over time do so because they feel better physically, psychologically, and interpersonally. In other words, they have found a waystation from the daily stressors of life. As these mind-body practices are usually done in groups, the person gains a sense of belonging and taps into the energy of the group.

There may come a point, as you train, where there is a nonjudgmental, peaceful awareness of being in the present and simply flowing along. Your sense of an individual, independent self has dropped off. Your mind is empty of your daily self-talk and mind wandering, and the subsequent agitation associated with these processes. Your mind has been stilled as you slowly flow along naturally. From the perspective of Zen Buddhism, this flowing along naturally is simply when you are hungry, you eat. When tired, you lie down. Your mind is empty and still when you eat. Your mind is empty and still when you lie down. Nothing else. Just eat. Just lie down. Whatever you are doing, just do that. Nothing else. So, when practicing tai chi or qigong, just practice tai chi or qigong. Nothing else. This is wuwei! This is ziran! This is being alive! Nothing else! [26]

Comparing the Effects Tai Chi and Qigong with Walking

Systematic reviews of research comparing tai chi exercise with walking in healthy adults, have reported positive effects of tai chi exercise on blood pressure, resting heart rate, stroke volume and cardiac output, lung capacity, and cardiorespiratory endurance, suggesting that tai chi benefits cardiorespiratory fitness.[27] A related meta-review suggested that in contrast to no exercise, tai chi and qigong provide significant but not robust benefits for hypertension (lowered diastolic and systolic blood pressure levels), and diabetes (lower homeostatic model assessment of insulin resistance and fasting blood glucose levels), both of which are linked with risk for

130

stroke.[28] Another study involving older women, compared tai chi exercise with a brisk walking group and a sedentary group in a 12-week intervention program. The results indicated that in comparison to the sedentary group, those who practiced tai chi 3-times a week for an hour showed enhanced maximal oxygen uptake (VO² max) and heart rate variability (i.e., spectral analysis of the duration of time intervals between heart beats). This same study also indicated greater nondominant knee extensor strength (the extensors are the muscles that straighten your leg) and single leg-stance time because of tai chi exercises in comparison to the brisk walking condition. Overall, this research suggests the practice of tai chi is an effective way to improve strength, balance, and flexibility.[29]

Research using Functional Magnetic Resonance Imaging (fMRI; a measure of brain activity) and involving older Chinese women, suggested the long-term effects of tai chi practice and walking on brain networks may differentially influence functional brain systems and brain plasticity. While not conclusive in suggesting a better or worse than comparison between tai chi and walking, this study encourages more research into how various physical training regimes may affect neurological connectivity and be used as a preventative strategy to counteract neurological deficits that occur later in life.[30]

Certainly, tai chi and qigong should be considered physical exercises that when practiced consistently provide beneficial neuropsychological and biophysical effects. It is also becoming clear too that incorporating tai chi and qigong into one's daily activities can have a long-lasting influence on well-being and happiness. Further, as we see people of all ages and abilities involved in the practice of tai chi and qigong, it should be noted that one is never too young nor too old, nor too mentally or physically impaired to take up these arts and find benefits. As Professor Santee also suggests, diligent practice of tai chi and qigong can bring harmony to mind and body, and a positive approach toward living.

Brief Treks to Deep Discovery

As Thoreau recognizes, our encounter with nature is just beyond the front door of our homes and apartments. Thus, when we consider brief treks, we recognize that we can have this type of adventure in our own neighborhoods or in areas that are close by where we live. It might be to engage like Euell Gibbons or Langdon Cook in their rambles to *Stalk the Wild Asparagus,* or other natural herbs and foods, or for an overnight camping experience.[31] Indeed, hiking in nature as one forages for natural herbs, or explores forests not visited before, or to sleep under the stars on an overnight camping trip, represent other artforms where we find pathways to encounter and connect with nature and ourselves in transformative ways. As Ed Brooker and Marion Joppe suggest, camping is an enjoyable activity that provides escape from urban living, with many opportunities for recreation and socialization.[32] Similarly, other research reports that the opportunity to be in nature, to learn outdoor skills and about the environment, and to be with others who share similar interests are strong motivating factors to partake in out-of-doors adventure experiences.[33] Nevertheless, there are barriers that some older adults might encounter that prevent this type of involvement, such as the physical ability to take on the ruggedness of the outdoors, finding peers who would also like to participate, and lack of resources (e.g., equipment, financial ability, Recreational Vehicle/trailer).[34]

If a camping expedition is not possible, however, visiting in a Blue or Green area is the next best thing. Blue areas are recognized places where people reach 100 years of age at rates 10 times greater than in the U.S. and have easy access to the natural environment.[35] Important health enhancing features of Blue areas include regular opportunity to be in nature, use of gardens to provide nutritious food, high involvement with families and others in the community, low stress, and living with purpose. Designated Blue areas include Sardinia, Italy; Loma Linda, California; Okinawa, Japan; Ikaria, Greece; and, Nicoya, Costa Rica. In contrast, Green areas are places characterized as diverse ecosystems, such as a forest, park, garden, or other natural areas where there is the existence of diverse vegetation. A brief trek into these natural areas is also suggested to have health benefits. Indeed, in research that explores Blue and Green areas for older adults, visiting a nearby park or natural area is suggested not only to provide an opportunity to get some fresh air, but also to enhance psychological well-being via feelings of renewal, restoration, and spiritual connection that are evoked by being in nature, as well as the opportunities for social exchange with family, friends, and others in the community.[36] Other research focusing on the exposure to nature has suggested that Green areas improve cognitive focus and concentration, impulse control, and the ability to delay gratification, as well as positive enhancement of self-esteem and mood.[37]

Furthermore, empirical research exploring the effects of brief treks into natural outdoor environments suggest many other benefits. For example, research involving participants from Spain, United Kingdom, Netherlands, and Lithuania that assayed exposure to Green areas suggested contact with natural outdoor environments to lower stress and enhance mental health.[38] Other related research, using a mobile electroencephalography (EEG) to record the emotional experiences of walkers in urban shopping, commercial and natural settings of Edinburgh, Scotland, found evidence suggesting higher meditation and lower frustration, as well as greater alertness and arousal while entering and moving through a Green space park.[39] Related research examining the effects of reflective garden-walking over a six-week duration, reported higher levels of self-reported quality of life and personal growth initiative at the end of the six-weeks.[40] Further, in a study that examined the benefits of reflective garden-walking for individuals with high psychological stress, post-test improvements were reported in individuals' levels of hopefulness, quality of life, and personal growth.[41] Other experimental research investigating the beneficial effects of Nordic hiking and climbing, indicated outdoor mountain hiking and climbing to significantly increase positive affect and activity, and lower anxiety and fatigue.[42] Overall, these studies collectively suggest exposure to Green spaces within urban settings lowers stress, enhances mood, and facilitates reflective activities that augment personal growth and quality of life. Further, the benefits of being in nature are so well recognized that it is suggested to be a form of medicine.[43]

Don't Be Afraid to Get Your Hands Dirty

Monty Don, a British horticulturist, writer, and broadcaster, is acclaimed world-wide for his gardening knowledge. Like the wisdom expressed in *The Jewel Garden: A Story of Despair and Redemption*, Monty Don espouses an approach to living that is oriented in the very rich humus of personal experience.[44] Sharing his story, Monty writes of difficult personal and business challenges, the anguish and life-shattering complications of depression, and how one's passion for living can be restored by a return to *terra firma* and gardening. Indeed, as Monty suggests, as a complement to medical therapies, toiling in the soil and working with the earth can itself be healing. A further realization of how horticulture therapy can be centering and restoring to the human spirit is also demonstrated in empirical research. For example, in a study summarizing the benefits of a gardening program for residents in low-income senior housing, participants reported that they chose to garden so as to reconnect with earlier times when they gardened, to be involved and learn something new, to be connected to beauty and growth, to be socially helpful in some manner, for mental health benefits, and to receive the end product of fruits and vegetables.[45] Similarly, in a review of horticulture therapy studies from 2008 to 2018 involving older adults, significant pretest-posttest improvements were noted on measures of anxiety, cognition, depression, physical well-being, quality of life and social relationships.[46] These findings again suggest the benefits of gardening, especially for those living in institutional environments. Other research has suggested that communal gardening may enhance older adults' sense of accomplishment, satisfaction, aesthetic pleasure, quality of life and emotional well-being, while expanding one's social network and combatting isolation.[47] Similarly, an experimental investigation exploring the benefits of a twelve-week horticultural therapy program for midlife women with affective disorder reports significant reduction in anxiety and depression symptoms, and enhanced self-esteem.[48] Another study involving nursing home residents in a weekly 60-minute horticulture activity for eight weeks, reported increased subjective happiness for both frail and prefrail nursing home residents taking part in the horticulture activity.[49] Other research has indicated gardening and horticulture therapy assists individuals in treatment of substance abuse and addiction, during inpatient psychiatric care, and as a prevention for pathologies related to lifestyles that involve sedentary and stressful jobs, insufficient physical activity, poor nutritional practice, and risk for substance abuse and addiction.[50]

Following Thoreau

As Thoreau noted, there is quite a bit to discover about nature as well as about ourselves when we walk. We can recount our past experiences and present concerns, and find new purpose and meaning in our lives. As the Covid-19 pandemic continued through 2021 and 2022, one author took on the task of taking a half-hour walk each day, through the parks and on the trails where he lived, for an entire year. In many ways, this regimen of daily walking is a test of one's mettle, but as Thoreau noted, also an opportunity to look deeply within.

It seemed rather unimaginable at first, to walk—day in, day out—for one whole year. At the start, even thinking about walking for 10 days in a row seemed rather implausible. With the recruitment of family members, though, a dedicated practice of walking everyday became a little easier to realize. Along the way too, there were many interesting occurrences, and moments of amazement. One interesting experience was just being outside every day—in the soft morning air, warming afternoon sunshine, as well as in the rain, cold and snow, and sun-scorched summer afternoons. Throughout the year we witnessed the changing seasons—from spring to summer, into fall, and later winter, and again spring. As various wildlife trails were explored, it was delightful to watch turtles bask in the sunshine on logs that jutted up from the pond where they lived. With wonder, we observed newly hatched ducklings as they followed their mother along the water's bank into the pond to begin their swimming lessons. We marveled to see and hear flocks of migrating birds as they flew through on their journey heading north or south. We observed changes in the trees as they awaken from winter, bloom in spring, and offer their fruit in late summer. We also discovered how the encouragement we gave one another bolstered our affect and helped us to continue our daily walks. We also sensed differences in ourselves; often observing a relaxing and shifting of mood as we hiked along. In a relaxed manner, we could then find insights into problems encountered in everyday living, and find ways to laugh at ourselves when we seemed to express trifling or inconsequent concerns. It was easy to realize that our daily walking was introducing a change in lifestyle—a change from a sedentary, desk-bound type of living, to one that was more active and immersed in the outdoors. We grasped that we did not just "think about exercising—yet never did it," as some folks may honestly report. Rather, we came to find great enjoyment in our walking. It was also interesting to encounter other hikers, who shared their comradery and posed thought-provoking questions. Our walks also provided us interesting things to tell others about. Walking early in the morning, as the sun first comes up and the dew or frost still lay on the ground, seemed to be the most exciting and invigorating time to walk—symbolically reminding us of the newness of each moment of the day, and sensing, as Professor Santee also noted with the practice of tai chi or qigong, "an awareness of flowing through the present."

Walking with Purpose: Life-Journey to Discovery and New Ways of Being

Throughout our life, we walk with purpose, moving along in our journey of becoming. The places where we have started, the challenges and people we met along the way, and the milestones passed, all mark the many moments of our personal transcendence. As Jungian analyst James Hollis suggests, frank and deep inner-reflection illuminates our past and leads us to live authentically.[51] Moreover, Hollis suggests by knowing ourselves more deeply, through the airing out and recognition of stumbling blocks and inner processes that have held us back, we may select and move onto "a path of enlargement," where without influence of the ego or external factors we may courageously live, directed by our own unique creed of personal values and beliefs.

Applying a chronological analysis, in a sense sketching out our "life-chart," where all the milestone events of our development are recognized and appraised in terms of their impact upon our personal growth, is one method to use that will help lead us into deeper reflection. Like the life story and reminiscence processes mentioned earlier, this mapping entails a life-review process that can begin to elucidate how we have changed, grown, and become throughout the life-course, and perhaps inspire us in some way as we take the next steps in our journey. In this type of sequential analysis, we might realize that our movement along our path has not been a straight line, but followed a course that has veered and turned at times, maybe even making a U-turn, or that we have come full circle in some ways. We can look deeper to find sources of joy and of despair that we have experienced in our life. If we detect repetition in thoughts and action that somehow prevent us from reaching our greatest potential, then we have a legitimate reason for making a "real-time" correction. We can seek to be more compassionate towards and accepting of ourselves and others. We can shift our thinking and acting to live a more fulfilled life. Like a written life-review, this type of life analysis provides opportunity for reflecting and connecting with others, talking about one's life, as well as finding insight into the dynamics of our living and legacy that we leave to others.[52]

Finding Awe in the Moment

A special technique of reflecting that can lead us to find awe in the moment is mindful walking. Using the skill of mindfulness and anchoring our attention to the present moment, in mindful walking we simply observe what thoughts arise as we make our way. Then without adding any judgment or clarifying our feelings, we let the thought pass. If we begin to dwell on a particular issue or thought, we can be gentle with ourselves, and not get caught up in the emotion or further amplification of any thought but to say, "just let it pass," and go on again. Walking with mindfulness allows us to become non-judgmental of others, to live without fear, and to dispel concerns about living up to our own, often unrealistic expectations.

Like reflective garden-walking, there has also been research examining the effects of mindful walking. For example, prewalk-postwalk survey research involving community-dwelling older adults indicated outdoor mindful walking twice a week for at least 30 minutes over the course of one month lowered negative affect measured at the post-walk survey.[53] In other research, middle-age and older long-distance walkers described walking much like a therapeutic process. That is, walking was an experience where they realize a calmness and a sense of capability as they consider life strains and challenging experiences.[54] Similarly, in a review of labyrinth walking, a type of reflective walking where one follows a path that curves or winds to create a geometric design (e.g., circle, square, rectangle, etc.), participants' often report positive thoughts, emotions, and sensations during and after their labyrinth walking.[55] Again, these findings suggest the positive psychological benefits of walking. So let us recognize walking as an "art." Like those who practice tai chi and qigong, journey on great treks, sail, go hiking through Green spaces, or stroll in a garden, we too may discover greater vitality and renewal in our living. Indeed, just as the actor who moves downstage and hits the center mark, our rambles into the outdoors can lead us to a deeper understanding of who we are—and as Thoreau suggests, we may encounter Nature's magnetism that will direct us "aright."

EIGHT — BUT THAT IS NOT HOW THE STORY ENDS: A RESPONSE TO THE COVID-19 PANDEMIC AND MOVING BEYOND

A favorite part of playing in a big band is watching couples as they dance. Looking out on the dance floor, it is satisfying to watch younger and older couples as they interact with one another by touch, glance, and movement. It is remarkable how they glide effortlessly past other couples as they dance. Such moments reflect the inner grace of these couples. In many ways, their dancing tells a story about their lives. On the dance floor are older couples, content with each other and the years spent together, and younger couples, equally graceful but full of expectation for the future. One learns much about people from playing at these dances. Here one can come to appreciate the challenges, frustrations, joys, and triumphs of our human interactions together.

Similarly, when we encounter illness in our dance of life, we meet new challenges and often learn about ourselves as we seek an understanding of our experience. Unquestionably, the Covid-19 pandemic has brought such a moment of challenge as we experienced and heard the tragic stories of life's disruption and heartbreaking loss of family members and friends. In this chapter, one of the authors discusses his involvement with a community band, the difficult tasks of adapting one's activities, and the struggle to breakout from the constraints imposed by the pandemic and stay involved in making music. We also identify ways music can be a form of coping, a way of meditation, an orientation of mindfulness, and ultimately become our personal and communal story.

When the Music and Dancing Stopped

Ballroom dancing is rather popular where I live in south-central Pennsylvania. It not only provides an opportunity to enjoy the benefits of a creative type of exercise, but also a way to engage with others and with the community. There are many dance clubs in the area where folks can go to dance. Moreover, several organizations exist where ballroom dancing occurs regularly and where one can find instruction in all types of ballroom dance, such as the foxtrot, tango, and waltz. Many couples I see on the dance floor are alumni of ballroom dance classes. One of the dance instructors in the area, a former military officer, gives regular classes on ballroom dancing. My wife and I are alumni of his classes (although, I admit I still dance with two left feet of which I tend to stare at when I dance). His instructions are memorable as he barked out the steps much like a drill instructor would training new recruits. Thus, I always recall his instructions: "Your left, your right, your left, your right, turn to your partner!" It is a somewhat unorthodox style of instruction, but again highly effective in that it still resonates with me as a guide to use the correct steps (although I still stare at my feet). But when the Covid-19 epidemic rampaged across the world, everything changed. Live music, dancing, and all forms of social gathering stopped. The big band I performed in had to curtail playing. No longer did we see 30 to 40 couples assemble together in the ballroom to learn the foxtrot or the tango. Most of the dance instruction classes continued online, if at all. The dance floor became empty and silent. Similarly, concerts, large and small clubs, and restaurants all had to cancel their presentation of music. In a music scene that was already struggling with local musicians finding less and less work even before Covid-19, the shutdown was devastating, and it was personal.

With the development of vaccines and boosters to address new variants, however, we are once again returning to life before the pandemic. Yet despite the breakthrough in developing the vaccines, people are still getting ill and dying. According to the World Health Organization Coronavirus Disease Dashboard, there are now over 600 million confirmed cases world-wide and over 6 million deaths due to Covid-19.[1] The United States of America alone has reported almost 100 million confirmed cases and over one million deaths due to the virus.[2] Moreover, we are now experiencing a triple-demic of Covid-19, flu, and respiratory syndromes.

Uneasy Transition

The chaos, uncertainty, and damage wrought over the last few years by Covid-19, indeed has thrust us into an uneasy transition from shutdown to a time of opening-up due to the availability of vaccines. We are reminded of a quote by Hans Anderson: "When words fail, sounds can often speak."[3] This quote can be interpreted that when we find things too hard to talk about, our feelings can be expressed in music. However, even this expression was threatened to be silenced during the pandemic.

At both personal and societal levels, the shutdown forced us to address how we would respond to the challenges of living during a pandemic. I was recently retired and looking forward to playing in the community band I enjoyed so much. I had been a member of the band for over 20 years, and was now idled by the pandemic. The challenge for me (and for many others) was that I no longer was able to enjoy playing music with my friends, and missed performing at concerts that I always looked forward to with excitement. I had many thoughts about the future of live music, and the dire prospect that we may not see it for a very long time. Not only that, but I was also concerned, as many were, about going out in public and attending social gatherings unless it was absolutely necessary (e.g., to doctors or other medical appointments). The result of this isolation for me was loss of contact with others. I reflected on my situation and tried to understand what was going on in other public performance groups, how others were handling being separated from doing what they loved, and what strategies were implemented to get through this horrible situation. As musicians, we all walked together in this experiential journey, thinking about the impact of the pandemic on older musicians, and how to stay creatively involved and keep the music alive.

Impact on Musicians and Public Performances: An End of the Community Band?

At the very beginning of the pandemic, we saw large ensembles stop all rehearsals and public performances. This response had impacted municipal bands and orchestras considerably. Once a mainstay of community involvement through its summer concerts, dances, and holiday performances, the music from town bands was silenced. We no longer saw an amphitheater packed with an audience waiting to hear a concert. Band members were forced to maintain an internally driven schedule of private practice, without the added incentive of weekly rehearsals and concerts where they could enjoy the comradery of fellow musicians, family, and friends. As we began to see the rollout of vaccines to provide protection from Covid-19, we were still unsure of the fate of our community bands. Could we entertain the possibility of the band's reappearance, although in some transformed way?

Many changes had to take place so we could still play and be safe. We had to understand what constituted good and bad practices regarding social distancing and mask wearing. We also had to consider the controversies surrounding these preventative health behaviors and vaccinations. During the pandemic when vaccines first became available, Covid-19 infection was affecting mostly the unvaccinated population. Also, at risk were children who were not old enough to receive a vaccination. The possible implications of how the pandemic would affect rehearsals and public performances involved whether large groups would still be able to perform together, or if some hybrid involving smaller ensembles, individual concerts, or duos and trios spaced well apart had to become the new norm. Other concerns involved how these concerts could be presented to an audience. Certainly, the pandemic caused inordinate stress and a great disruption to our lives. We lost beloved family members and friends, and felt separated from others in our community. But, if there ever could be a silver lining, perhaps it is what we learned about ourselves: The great need we have to be socially connected, to contribute to our community, and to find adaptive and innovative ways of continuing our daily musical practice and ensemble rehearsals.

Playing and Listening: Good, Questionable, and Bad Distancing

When the weather is fine, it is easier to conduct rehearsals and performances outdoors with a larger group, as one can establish safe social distancing between band members. However, as concerts were required to be moved indoors due to weather, safety concerns became more problematic. During the pandemic, several university stage-bands used a combination of plexiglass shields (often surrounding each member), well-spaced distancing, and mask-wearing. Masks were worn when not playing a horn, for instance, but put in place during break or rests. Also, masks were available that had an opening cut in them to provide access to mouthpieces. Bell covers were also available. Other issues such as the size of the ensemble and how many musicians could gather safely together had to be considered. We can think of an example where a community band or orchestra restarts rehearsals but instead of the usual 50 pieces is now reduced to around 10 members. Here, one could ensure that proper distancing, masking, shield wearing, and or plexiglass are in place. It was also recommended that all members play in the same direction (i.e., not in a circular configuration where members would be facing each other) to avoid aerosol being spread to other members. However, even with these precautions, there were significant concerns that involve how one's personal sense of safety is affected, who gets to rehearse, how members are contacted and chosen for rehearsal, and what is the future standing of those who either voluntarily opt out or were never made aware of their options due to communication problems.

Musicians' Response

Throughout the pandemic, musicians were very creative in establishing methods to stay safe and to present their music to the public. We saw and continue to see presentations on *YouTube,* and other video formats such as *Zoom,* where musicians can perform and display their artistry. With the expansion of social media, contact with other musicians and the public can now occur via *Facebook, TikTok, Spotify,* and *Instagram* to name a few. My response during the pandemic, and something I continue to do, was to make videos of my own playing, and to share them with another friend and musician. We produced remote videos of our parts individually, and then exchanged them to be mixed and presented on social media (e.g., *YouTube* and *Facebook*). At the height of the pandemic, in-house performances in restaurants and other venues were non-existent. But with expected loosening of restrictions due to the new vaccines, we began to see limited live performances at these venues. The intriguing questions musicians had to consider were, how would the listening public react to these approaches? Will these modifications and restrictions affect attendance? How long can a performer hold audience interest in say a constant diet of *YouTube* concerts? As a matter of survival, many musicians presented online concerts with a link for the viewer to send money to the performer. During the pandemic, many of us found comfort in the music the performers shared online and were inspired by the collective hope and way of staying socially connected that the music offered. The pandemic also gave rise to new live music-streaming companies, and other industries pivoted and made adjustments that are now permanent.[4]

When we consider "virtual" or "online" performances, one issue is the attention span of the average listener. For example, some of us can only watch or listen to about 20 seconds of a video presentation before we lose interest and begin to look for something else. It is not uncommon for folks to report that they constantly bounce from one video to the next, without watching and listening to the very end. One can speculate that possibly it is the social experience itself, as well as various distractions that curiously keep our attention during a public performance. For example, in live concerts or in-the-park performances, one can watch other aspects of the situation such as other people or the scenery, and then be drawn back into the performance. Such additional background stimulation may not be available in online performances. Furthermore, vigilantly staring at a computer screen or smartphone can be very draining on one's attention span, and no doubt contributes to the seeking and constant clicking to find new videos as a substitute for the more natural distractions found in a live performance.

Research on Droplets, Aerosols, and Band Instruments

As described earlier, musicians are concerned about personal health and safety when playing music with others. For example, singing is recognized as being very problematic, as it involves the production of aspirated and unaspirated speech sounds, the former of which release a higher concentration of aerosols into the surrounding area.[5] Thus, choir rehearsals have been particularly singled out as super-spreader events. When we consider ways to stay safe, perhaps the most drastic prevention response is not to sing or play music at all. More practically, however, proper distancing between ensemble members and refraining from sharing microphones with others seem to be more reasonable safe practices. To understand this concern more, data on the transmission of aerosols and droplets from wind and brass instruments were gathered in various research studies.[6] One investigation on wind and brass instruments and their aerosol production was conducted by Ruichen He and colleagues.[7] Key factors contributing to the risk of spreading airborne viruses are aerosol concentration, size of the aerosol particles, and flow rate of particles. Other transmission concerns include particle release through keyholes, embouchure holes, and instrument bells as one plays a wind or brass instrument. Measuring these factors, aerosol generation was found to be the lowest in tubas. Tubas produced aerosol concentrations lower than that found in normal breathing and speech. An intermediate level of risk is found in bassoons, piccolos, flutes, bass clarinets, French horn, and clarinet. These instruments produced aerosol concentrations comparable to that found in normal breathing and speaking. Finally, of the 10 instruments reviewed, trumpets, oboes, and bass trombones produced more aerosols than found in normal breathing or speaking. Important caveats presented by these researchers that provide direction for future research, are differences in the performing styles of musicians, reed selection (i.e., width, hardness) for woodwind instruments, blowing pressure, and ambient air flow and room ventilation. A yet unanswered question concerns the volume and risk of condensation material emitted when using a spit valve as well as the amount of water that pools on the floor or spit mat. Obviously, distancing is important. The Centers for Disease Control (CDC) guidelines recommended six feet between individuals. Although in some instances the distancing guidelines have been adjusted to three feet. The use of plexiglass panels placed between members is another way to reduce risk of exposure. However, care must be used as these shields could interfere with the room's HVAC system's ability to effectively change out the air in the room.[8] Many of these guidelines are also recommended for music therapists when working with their clients.[9]

Workable Protocols

Music organizations continue to have in place quite excellent safety protocols following CDC guidelines. Community bands post and try to adhere to the precautions and rules for how rehearsals should be conducted.[10] It should be noted that these safety procedures predate vaccines but may again be revisited because of a rise of new variants. One consideration is that the number of ensemble members gathering together should be proportional to the size and capacity of the room. Larger rooms can accommodate more people than smaller rooms, provided that appropriate Covid-19 protocols are in place. Other concerns include the use of face masks and bell covers for wind instruments, and with the face masks having only a hole placed in it to accommodate a mouthpiece. Other preventative practices include the checking of body temperatures and asking "Covid-19 related" questions to screen members as they enter the rehearsal or performance site. Interestingly, some protocols stipulate rehearsal breaks be taken with the front and back doors of the rehearsal area propped open to allow air flow to "air out" the space. Importantly, a log should be maintained documenting all activities occurring within the facility, the people in attendance, and all areas that need to be disinfected.

The Older Musician

Although the pandemic impacted people of all ages, it is not surprising that older musicians were at greater risk for and experienced more comorbid illness and complications due to Covid-19 than their younger counterparts. Some of the physical outcomes of the Covid-19 virus included changes in respiratory function, paresis/paralysis of the laryngeal nerves, and possible permanent lung damage.[11] Certainly, damage to the vocal cords and lungs also impairs one's ability to sing or play a wind or brass instrument. The concomitant psychological consequences of this impairment may include increases in stress, anxiety, and sadness. Further, when illness is encountered, the older musician may express and experience a form of grief associated with being separated from the ensemble and its members. Other factors that impact the well-being of many older musicians are cancelled rehearsals and performances, and an unfamiliarity with using new technology to stay musically engaged. A particularly disheartening outcome is the fear that during a quarantine or any separation from their musical community, the older musician may not have the opportunity to play or sing with others again in their lifetime.[12] And, indeed, during the pandemic, many musicians experienced very negative emotions such as "desperation, existential anxiety, and panic."[13]

Keeping the Music Alive

The pandemic disrupted many things in our lives, one of which is a regular and routine practice schedule. One of the more important features of learning and playing music is to develop an effective routine that contains strategies toward becoming successful in our practicing, rehearsing, and public performances. Even if one is a stay-at-home, garage, or basement performer, staying motivated and engaged in one's music is challenged by events like the pandemic. We continue to hear folks say: "I find it hard to practice at the same level pre-pandemic," or "My interest in playing has severely diminished," and unfortunately some have given up making music all together. Certainly, these types of responses to the pandemic reflects something going on in our deeper psychology. We understand that for many, the pandemic was a soul-changing event. The result of which was a diminished interest in life, uncertainty about the future, feeling overwhelmed, and an inability to find a way to cope or a way out of the pandemic. Perhaps at a more mundane level, we can understand how our motivation, enthusiasm, and engagement may lag, particularly when we cannot engage in the same way as before the pandemic.

147

The performing musician thrives on playing at clubs, being with others at concerts, and rehearsing with friends or bandmates. Thus, when these opportunities no longer exist, musicians feel a threat to their identity and sense of purpose.

Furthermore, there are other reasons older musicians became unmotivated during the pandemic. We may have felt overwhelmed when family members and friends became sick, or died from Covid-19. We may have feared that we too would become infected, preventing us from engaging with others in our community as we once did. Another reason is that we can become inundated by all the health news—positive and negative— surrounding new cases and variant forms of Covid-19. When vaccines first became available, many people felt frustration trying to schedule a vaccine for oneself or others. We now see more vaccines available than people eligible to take them. It is also important to mention that we may no longer have the "triggers" available that inspire us to stay focused in our musical routines— such as regular rehearsal and playing schedules. These also influence our intrapersonal and interpersonal approach to music. For the listener, a regular menu of in-the-park performances and concerts can keep us engaged. For the musician, perhaps we have quit practicing because we cannot find a way to structure our personal practice sessions to be constructive, and perhaps feel we are simply running over the same old material and not making any headway. This is a particularly common challenge in our everyday practicing, even without living through a pandemic. Christine Carter proposes that one reason musicians feel they are not making progress in their practice, and importantly why their hard work during practice does not translate necessarily into a good public performance, is how we structure our practice sessions. One simple strategy to improve our performance that she proposes is to alter the way we practice. An effective alteration is to change from the rather conventional "blocked" practice schedule, to a "random," or "interweaved" practice schedule. A blocked practice schedule is where we might learn a musical phrase by repeating it until mastered before moving on to the next section or passage in the piece. She cites that this approach is good for practice but may not transfer well to a performance. One reason is that we can become bored with playing and our mind is no longer as active as it processes information. In contrast, random, or interweaved practice, she proposes, transfers better to real performance situations as it allows the mind to remain active. This type of practice involves interspersing and moving around different components, or phrases of the musical piece. For example, we can learn in order phrase 1 (p1), then phrase 2 (p2), then phrase 3 (p3), and so on, but then begin to intersperse them in a random way (e.g., p1, p3, p2; p2, p1, p3, and so on).[14] Of course, the failure to maintain a practice schedule and subsequent failure to progress becomes exacerbated by changes in health. As many have experienced, managing health concerns, making Doctor appointments, and traveling to see caregivers can become so burdensome that one can find little time for much else, let alone practicing and staying engaged with their craft.

Realistic Goals

One way to continue to be engaged in one's music making is to take a hard look at our goals, and to make adjustment when needed. Conventional wisdom and psychology principles propose that instead of trying to achieve broad or undefined goals, or to attain something very daunting (e.g., to learn all Charlie Parker solos), we first should set specific and attainable short-term goals. For example, my goals are to memorize all the pieces that make up my jazz duo's performance playlist, and to also learn as many "standards" as possible. But to avoid becoming overwhelmed by these goals, I might set for myself the goal of trying to learn one song per week instead of engaging in a marathon session. And, as I learn a new song, add it to the performance playlist that I want to memorize. Also, it is important to have an action plan. Research shows that having a clearly articulated plan of action to achieve one's goal, leads to its successful attainment.[15] In addition, having a social support network is vitally important. This network only needs to consist of the one person you find most important in your life to help you achieve your goals.[16] Similarly, when planning a successful practice routine, one can identify the particular goals to try to achieve in each practice session, the length of the session, and an evaluation of the session. For example, Yo-Yo Ma stated that he worked on a piece of music by learning one measure a day. He relates that at the age of four, he started out by learning Bach Cello Suites one measure at a time.[17] Now for some that may be fine-tuning it a bit too much, but the point is that often one must take many small steps to reach their goal. So, to learn a piece of music during a particular rehearsal session, the best practice is to work on one section or phrase at a time. When that is learned well, then move to another section or phrase. Then move toward an interspersed practice format. Regarding the length of the sessions, it is suggested that a shorter rather than longer practice session is most effective. Again each session should be tailored in a particular way by the individual to assist them in their goal attainment, with a good rule of thumb to have the session go no more than 20 to 30 minutes before taking a break. Finally, it is important to evaluate your rehearsal. Did you reach the goal you expected? Were you trying to do too much? Not enough? Another way to stay engaged with your musical practice is to periodically evaluate your equipment. Do you have a good set of strings on your guitar or violin? Are your pads in shape on your clarinet, flute, or sax? Are your brass instrument's valves and tubing in good order? If you are fortunate enough to own a lot of musical equipment, it can be refreshing to "rediscover" equipment that might be in storage or has not been played recently.

Another hinderance to staying involved in your musical practice is perfectionism. Not only do we live in an imperfect world, but events like the pandemic and other negative events emphasize disruption, chaos, and imperfection. There is an old joke that a genii granted a mandolin player (substitute instrument of your choice) two wishes. The mandolin player asked for world peace. The genii said that was too hard, and to ask for something else. The mandolin player then asked, "well I would like to play in tune." The genii then said, "what was your first wish again?" Another mandolin joke I believe attributed to Tim O'Brien is that tuning a mandolin is like achieving world peace. It will never happen, but one should keep trying. The point is that one should strive to play as well as one can and as close to being in tune as possible, but to believe that you should expect to have the "perfect" performance or practice session is setting yourself up for defeat. The key is to be reasonable.

Music as Coping

The above discussion about goal setting and action plans alludes to how we might cope under stress. Research suggests that we can engage in two types of coping: problem-focused and emotion-focused coping.[18] With problem-focused coping we can approach stress as a problem to be solved. Following this approach, one can engage in active planning such as establishing a practice/rehearsal protocol, determining length of time, and when, where, and how to practice or rehearse. We found that having a good action plan results in success in achieving one's goals.[19] Emotion-focused coping helps one to endure, reduce, or alleviate stress by such techniques as meditation, prayer, or venting of emotions. Problem-focused and emotion-focused coping techniques often overlap with each other. We may create a plan (problem-focused) that dovetails with an emotion-focused strategy. For example, we may plan to listen to 30 minutes of music per day to help us relax.

Music as Meditation

One coping strategy we propose is to use music as meditation. Using this type of strategy, we suggest that as you play your instrument you do not think about what you are playing. Rather, as you play a stringed instrument for example, just let your fingers simply go where they want to go. If playing a wind or brass instrument, again just let your fingering wander and play in whatever register the instrument takes you. The point made here is to make music free of any preconceived expectations. That is, kind of like being on "automatic pilot," you do not consciously think about what you are doing and for that matter do not even monitor what you are playing. In this type of meditative practice, let your mind become blank, and try not to see, hear, or attend to what you are playing, but rather just play and let the music create and express itself.

151

Music as Mindful Playing

The practice of mindfulness is to direct one's attention to what is happening in the moment. Mindfulness can involve focusing just on one's breathing, so as to avoid distractions such as ruminating on the past or worrying about the future.[20] In this style of practice we use the technique of mindfulness to help us refine our playing. In this manner, as one plucks or sounds a note or musical phrase, one's attention is directed to the playing and the shaping of the musical idea. One listens to the tone, quality of sound, register, pitch, not in an analytic way or in a critical way, but in a way where one is aware of being in the presence of playing that note or making an artistic expression. Mindful playing allows you to experience each note as its own important contribution toward attaining closer contact to one's music, instrument, sense of self, and the audience.

A Broader Interpretation

We have proposed that ways to continue to remain engaged with one's music includes setting realistic goals in practice and performance situations, and in assessing one's progress. We have also suggested that music can be used as a coping mechanism, to help us through the stressful and difficult times in our lives. Further, we note that music can be used as meditation as well as an act of mindfulness. These proposals can be folded into a broader life-view or perspective that incorporates the following guiding principles.[21]

In order to live a life that is fulfilling and hopeful then, we should first and foremost not be afraid to live our life. This fearless approach to living is embodied in four ideas: First, we should engage in our daily living as one would engage in play. As we see children playing, we can appreciate their ability to fully engage in the moment and become fully immersed in the activity. Second, to play is also an act of creation. As we play, we let go of our self-awareness that can lead to self-doubt and self-criticism that can thwart our creativity. Third, we withhold judgment. Not only do we refrain from judging others but most importantly we do not overly judge ourselves. Fourth, and above all, we should have fun and create without fear. We can only create when we boldly go forward unafraid and throw off the fetters of judgment and recrimination. A common wisdom involving creativity is that one cannot create or be attuned to one's muse when under stress, or in an environment where others may judge you or when you are overly critical of yourself. Thus, through music, and more broadly through any of our creative expressions, we understand that an art-filled way of living is a way of evolving and creating a synthesis that integrates the many challenges we will meet and overcome, as well as the new adventures we undertake. Through our music and involvement in other arts we can achieve a new orientation that impacts us cognitively, behaviorally, and emotionally. In essence, when we harness our creativity, we think about, act toward, and feel about our life, others, and the world in a way that transforms us and truly opens us up to a celebration of life.

Music as Story: Facing the Challenges of Later Life

We invite the reader to consider how musical works also express a story. Here is a thought experiment to try: Find and listen to a recording of a song that you enjoy. As you listen, consider what effect the music has on your thinking and feelings? Is the music uplifting, inspiring, or relaxing in any way? As you consider the lyrics of the song, what insights into yourself or another person does the music uncover? After listening, did you sing or hum parts of the melody? Was your mood affected? Did it make you feel happy, melancholy? Did it renew you in some way that helped you meet the challenges of the day? Each of us will hear the music and the song lyrics in our own way. What we think and how we feel when we hear John Lennon and Paul McCartney's song "A Little Help from My Friends," or Queen's "We are the Champions," will be different for people of different backgrounds and generations. We experience the world from our own point of view, from our own lens of understanding. This perceptual self-lens frames and directs our thoughts and actions and reflects our personal quirks, foibles, idiosyncrasies, and deeper psychological motives and concerns. Thus, in listening to music we also may discover a story about ourselves, find new self-understanding, and gain insight into the challenges that lie ahead.

Save the Last Dance for Me: A Postscript

In the previous sections we considered some of the effects of living through a pandemic. As we move forward beyond the pandemic, important implications for how we stay healthy are of concern. During the pandemic, initially vaccines were rolled out in stages with essential personnel receiving the vaccine first, then folks in nursing homes and retirement centers, followed by those at risk because of underlying health conditions, and then by others to produce a "herd" immunity. Now an assortment of vaccines are readily available, along with boosters and other medicines if one becomes sick. Further, the Centers for Disease Control (CDC) are continually updating guidelines for best practices for older adults. Learning from the pandemic, it is recognized that being current in vaccination or taking the precaution to use a mask just makes good sense.[22] Unfortunately, vaccines and mask-wearing, two effective and well-known public health behaviors practiced world-wide, have become politicized. Groups of anti-vaxxers and anti-maskers are confronting (sometimes violently) common-sense protocols regarding a very wide range of health practices. School board members are threatened by the public when they vote to put mask mandates for schools in place. Some politicians have gone so far as to recommend criminal sanctions on public health officials who "force" that masks should be worn in schools and other public places. These issues will intensify if it again becomes necessary to impose a health quarantine or adopt restrictive mask wearing requirements. However, the good news is that at present, there are currently no Covid-19 restrictions regarding social contact for vaccinated persons, and community bands now can play together without masks or social distancing provided members are vaccinated.

Personal Post, Postscript: The Battle Continues

The big band I play with is now rehearsing and performing "live" once again. We are all excited to play to a live audience. Our rehearsals initially were held outside in mild weather, and with bell covers and face masks used when inside. Now we can practice and perform without masks because of the vaccine. The rollout of vaccines has been aggressive and in no small part contributed to the opening of community parks and other venues. We are beginning to come out of our basements and have reduced the number of *Zoom* meetings in favor of "face-to-face" contact. Those who are fully vaccinated can forego masks in many situations. Although common sense as well as state and local stipulations are to be followed, fully vaccinated people can essentially do all those things they did pre-pandemic. The development and rollout of vaccines have allowed children and grandchildren to visit their grandparents without fear of spreading Covid-19. We can again join and sing in choirs. We can now attend our places of worship. We can visit family and friends who we have not seen in such a long time. Also, as a testament to our resilience as musicians, during the lockdown, many reported that it gave them a chance to investigate new creative techniques, to learn new technologies, and to think outside the box. Many musicians learned how to maintain connections with their peers, but also reported initiating new collaborations, thus preserving social interactions and advancing in the creative process.[23] Indeed, there are many things we learned from the pandemic. Certainly, one is a feeling that we have become reborn in some way. However, this feeling must also be tempered by a sense of uncertainty about other viral threats, and other questions about how safe are we really?[24] For example, many other viruses associated with respiratory illness and flu are on the rise and pose a threat, especially to those already compromised by other illness concerns (e.g., pulmonary disorder, heart disease, diabetes).

Although the United States moved rapidly in getting as many people fully vaccinated as possible, there is still much vaccine hesitancy. This reticence can be attributed to many factors, political, personal, and social. Members of the music community have advocated that everyone should become vaccinated. And musical artists such as Clint Black, John Legend, and Latin artists, such as Gloria Trevi, and Chayanne have joined in and added their voices to promote vaccine awareness.[25] Yet, many parts of the world are still falling short of vaccines and medicines for many diseases. The resulting world-wide health crisis we see now is in part due to inability to acquire sufficient vaccines to reach herd immunity, poverty that limits and constrains developing countries, their governments and people, and corporations that limit production of key medicines or outsource production and use cheaper or unregulated ingredients, all of which affect appropriate disease prevention and care.[26] The United States has become a leader in distributing its excess supply of vaccines to areas of the world needing it most. Thus, as we know, the war can be won, but the battle is not over.

Like those in war zones, we are confronted with the devastation and loss of lives due to Covid-19. The pandemic has taken millions of lives worldwide and over one million Americans have died because of Covid-19. And, in many places the pandemic is not yet under control.[27] Further, everyone has known someone who became sick or died from Covid-19, and much like those who have survived a battle in wartime, also experience some form of Post-Traumatic Stress. We feel we are coming out of the rubble of a war caused by Covid-19 and has left us with a profound sickness of the soul. But make no mistake, we are still in a war. We must be vigilant of new variants, as well as regional and seasonal surges. These concerns are further compounded by the occurrence of other strains particularly among people who are not yet or refuse to get vaccinated. In addition, some scientists are proposing that Covid-19 will remain endemic in the population. That is, like the flu, it will always be present. The disturbing realization we must face is how many lives lost will society find acceptable due to Covid-19 each year.

Finally, we must consider what we have lost. Each of our reported experiences and feelings are often interrelated and felt at different levels of intensity. We mentioned the loss of family, friends, and loved ones during this pandemic. The hole that is created by any death is something that is never filled. The grief one feels, while perhaps moderating in its intensity, is one that is always experienced and forever a part of one's life. Also, reported by many is the loss of their faith or their religion. When the pandemic shutdown was at its most pronounced, churches, synagogues, mosques, and other places of worship were closed. Attempts to provide online services were met with varying degrees of success and failure, with many folks not tuning in and not watching. Many are now making the decision whether to go back to their place of worship or have lost their faith entirely because of this pandemic. Another reported loss is the loss of intimacy one has with one's partner. Contributing factors could be anxiety surrounding contracting the virus, job loss, stress of maintaining homelife with online work, and the addition of teaching children at home. Disturbingly, rates of domestic violence and child abuse have risen dramatically. Also, our involvement with and connection to others through participation in and attendance at community and other events, as well as visits with family and friends have been disrupted. In fact, many report a general loss of connection to others and a disruption of the continuity of life as a result of the pandemic. Loss of work, loss of enjoyable activities, loss of contact with others may have had a direct effect on peoples' report of a general lack of interest in doing the things they once found enjoyable. Although one can hope—and there is a hope—that as a result of the pandemic we will learn better about how to care for one another, how to share our resources more equitably, and how to live in harmony. But again, we also know that this hope must be tempered with the sober remembrance of those we have lost and those we will still lose to this disease. As we begin again to take to the dance floor, to sing, and to make music, we must also make the commitment that through these activities we remember and celebrate those whose lives have been lost.

When we think of resilience, the following terms come to mind: overcoming, endurance, persistence, recovery, bouncing back, elasticity, adaptation, and growth. However, other views of resilience portray it as something that is defined by its endpoint, in that you have overcome the challenge, learned, adapted, or beat the odds. We are also given suggestions such as keeping a sense of purpose, maintaining positive relationships, being hopeful, learning from your mistakes, and accepting change, to name a few. As one person puts it, resilience means that "even when you feel you are at the end of your tether, you still find a way to continue on." We can further include concepts such as recovery, adaptation, and persistence when we think of what it means to be resilient. Recovery implies that we have met the challenge, learned from it, and now see a sense of purpose realized from the adversity. Adaptation implies that we have modified how we now approach life. Persistence dictates that we persevere in the face of daunting odds.

Nonetheless, life is full of many challenges. We all experience trials and tribulations, feel pain, stumble, fall, are hurt, angered, frustrated, and at times become outraged. Often, the challenges we face are ongoing with seeming little end or bright future in sight. For some, they may endure a debilitating, life-long illness, or experience grief over the loss of a loved one that is so profound that they feel it unbearable. Indeed, there are numerous struggles in life, and we will fall many times. Yet instinctively, we will seek to rise to our feet again. As a Japanese proverb expresses, "...fall seven times, stand up eight." However, we propose there is more to being resilient than simply getting back up when one falls. Often getting back up can be a long process, requiring us to reorient and change our patterns of living while we also deal with other life concerns. Moreover, as we pass through midlife into older age, we encounter many challenges. We will experience illness, death of friends and loved ones, discriminations, and social injustices. Often, it might seem like we are fighting a battle that we can never win. Thus, our perceptions of these events can lead us to feel hopeless and that our lives and the world have no meaning. How then does one continue the fight in the face of insurmountable odds? We propose that to be resilient is to understand that adversity presents an existential threat to who we are and our continue personal growth as a human being. Further, when we comprehend that adversity and the threat it presents go hand in hand, we have gained the insight needed to adaptively respond and move onto the path of resilience.

In this chapter, we embrace a qualitative approach toward understanding resilience. That is, we hope to offer for discussion various characteristics we may attribute to someone whom we deem a resilient person. Further, we recognize these characteristics reflect and include the creative and artful processes that underlie our efforts to cope effectively and surmount life's challenges. Thus, in accord with similar conceptualizations, we propose that one way to describe personal growth, resilience, and becoming throughout the life course is as a process of metamorphosis.[1] A metamorphosis is a transformation, a change from what one was, to what one is now and what they are becoming. We note though, that we never really complete this process of becoming. Instead, we continuously engage in what we will call a metamorphic resilience. Metamorphic resilience is an amending and improving action. It is the result of a self-realizing process in which we become aware of our existential fears (i.e., extinction, mutilation, loss of autonomy, separation, and ego death), as well as darker aspects of our unconscious mind (e.g., anger, biases, impulses, repressions).[2] Coupled with these new insights, metamorphic resilience directs us to hold onto hope and seek pathways to new ways of being.[3] Thus, it embodies a personal growth that not only contains common assumptions of resilience, such as recovery, adaptation, and persistence, but also a subtle belief that in our confrontations with adversity and life-challenges, we can "rise like a phoenix" to "rebuild and renew" ourselves.[4] From this orientation, we may effectively meet and overcome life's difficulties, and adaptively move beyond how we may have lived and operated in the past. To further understand what metamorphic resilience means, we consider those qualities that give us the courage and confidence to overcome adversity and grow as a person. In doing so, we submit that a metamorphic resilience is imbued with three qualities: The Existential Stance, Creativity, and Living Story.

The Existential Stance

Challenge and adversity bring into sharp focus the duality of our lives. This duality is exemplified in the existential idea of liminal space. Liminal space is that in-between space — that place of transition between living and dying, fellowship and isolation, health and illness, and joy and sorrow. This transitory, in-between space threatens the status quo of our existence. We are faced with who we were, a person not confronted with these challenges, to who we are now, a person who now must live with those challenges. The trials and tribulations we experience within this liminal space represent an existential threat to who we are, what we will become, and what we must resolve. We can utilize a variety of coping techniques to address the difficulties before us. These coping strategies can take the form of actively trying to resolve our concerns. For example, we can approach the threat as a problem to solve. We can gather more information, seek the help of others and create a plan to deal with our situation. Along with these instrumental ways of facing and working with our challenges, we can also deal with the threat we face by managing our emotional response. For example, to minimize the threat we may use prayer or meditation to modulate our feelings, or we can just change our feelings by accepting or denying the threat. We may do other things as well, such as exercising or taking a walk to "clear our head." Whatever coping technique we adopt, the intention is that it will help us move beyond the discomfort and uneasiness of our current situation and the stress we are experiencing. However, this is not a simple process. As one grows older, there is an ever-increasing awareness of the impermanence and finiteness of one's life, and perhaps too an awareness of one's ability to live independently or to act freely. Other existential challenges may arise as we may feel past our prime in some way, or feel unappreciated or devalued by society or others, and struggle to see ourselves in a positive light.

Becoming aware of these existential challenges is the first step in initiating an adaptive response that leads us to find a path to creativity and fulfillment in our older age. Thus to engage in this adaptive and fulfilled way of living, we must hold an existential stance of overcoming and seek effective ways to respond to the challenges in our lives. We propose that one existential stance with which we are endowed and may utilize is that of the warrior.

The Warrior Mindset

The warrior mindset is to take the stance of a fighter. Much like the character Rocky Balboa in the film *Rocky*, seemingly overmatched and against all odds, one continues to struggle and persevere. This mindset seizes on the conflict between living a life of meaning, against a background of what we see as the meaninglessness of our world. Thus, the warrior mindset adopts the motivational posture of "I may not win the battle, but I will persist and stay in the fight." It is not a nihilistic vision, but rather one where we boldly strive to become the creator of our own fate. It is in this willful act of holding hope for our desired outcome, that our living becomes meaningful. The warrior mindset also goes beyond concepts of heroic acts, or heroism. It is not defined by the outcome or the person, but instead is an all-encompassing way to approach the many challenges in life. It reflects an inner drive to overcome and continue despite the hardships we might face. Other important acts of the warrior mindset is to summon the courage to face our fears, to pursue an inner truth, to express a personal humility, and to endure and carry on. Thus, we fight because there is something noble worth fighting for; believing in the cause we take up, and discerning value in our efforts to enact positive change.

To take on the mindset of a warrior is to act with purpose, even if it means to act alone. To act alone does not mean to live separately from or in opposition towards others. We all share similar fears, challenges, and adversity. But to act alone in this context is to understand that comparing one's state to those of others is not productive. We constantly make social comparisons that establish how we are doing compared to others. These comparisons are designed to emphasize our differences in relation to others and how we measure up or fail to measure up in society. We may think of upward social comparisons where, concerned with our ego, we compare ourselves to someone in a better state than we are, or downward social comparisons, where we compare our present state to someone worse than us. A common downward social comparison story is where we hear of the person who complains of having no shoes until meeting a person with no feet. This story implies many things, one of which is that we should be thankful for what we have when we compare our state to those who have very little. A downward social comparison may make us feel better, but perhaps also instills a "feeling of guilt" that perhaps portrays in some way a personal conceit or disdain for having more than those less fortunate. In contrast, an upward social comparison to those better off than us might motivate us to strive toward achieving something better but may also illuminate in very stark terms our deficiencies that we will never be able to overcome. We propose that social comparisons, upward or downward, have rather limited meaning for us when we confront life's existential challenges. Comparing oneself to another does little to address the challenge and how one will respond. We propose that the process and resultant outcomes of social comparisons, like checking a box on a checklist of personal accomplishments or keeping a "life" score, are myths that further perpetuate the illusion that we are different from others and that others are different from us. The warrior mindset then is a critical feature of metamorphic resilience, in that this orientation compels us to see our challenges and situation realistically. In our view, to embrace this outlook is to take on the role of the creator in shaping our understanding of life-challenges, of participating meaningfully in communal roles and relations, and in finding joy and celebration in our living.

Creativity

The process of creating is the second quality of metamorphic resilience. A creative mindset gives the individual the latitude to overcome life's challenges and to work to bring about resolution. A creative mindset recognizes that difficult tasks in life are only challenges, and each setback or failure is a new learning opportunity. In effect, we are only limited in becoming who we were meant to be by what we have not yet been able to imagine. Thus, as the artist creates and affects change through their art, the act of creating brings us novel ways to imagine our world, find new perspective to our situation in life, and provides us a different context that elicits continued growth.

Indeed, whether it is through painting, ceramics, singing, dancing, or other arts, the act of creating is to bring into existence something new, something unique. It offers a catharsis that frees our emotions and spurs an inner insight that aids us in enacting positive change and finding resolution to our problems.[5] The product created, whether a sculpted vase, painting, song, or new activity in our everyday living, now symbolically portrays and conveys a new sense of purpose and meaning for our lives. It transcends all concepts of time and space in that this work of art may now speak to each person in a very different way. Just as Bob Ross, the famous PBS painter often remarked, there are no mistakes in painting, just wonderful creative accidents. We add that our creative approach to life's challenges can often be full of mistakes. However, in many ways our assumption of what is a mistake is not determined by what others impose on us, but rather what we impose on ourselves. Each step and each accomplishment, however lacking or meager in some way, whether a "mistake" or "success," signifies and thus is worthy of respect and appreciation for how the person is growing. It is in the act of creating that we transcend concepts of self-abrogation, failure or success. Indeed, in our "mistakes," those happy little accidents, we gain insight and experience a transformation in our living. Accordingly, our creativity guides us to be resilient in our life orientation. However, the act of creation is difficult and messy. The muse does not give of itself easily. But a creative approach to living seeks to embrace and overcome challenge by allowing the individual the freedom to fashion solutions, resolve dissonance, and move beyond failing or succeeding.

Living Story

Our lives are a story. The third quality of metamorphic resilience is the realization that you are the creator of your life story. As author then, you have the freedom to embrace themes of self-discovery, depict scenes of deep personal meaning, and portray plots that allow you to examine and proclaim your life purpose, as well as the liberty to pursue alternative and different endings to the many chapters of your life. Metamorphic resilience is having the options to embrace an optimistic outlook and attitude, to direct your thinking in a way that recognizes and avoids the negative and illogical premises that lead to false and unproductive conclusions, to plot your own course, and, as much as is possible, to direct your life and your personal story of becoming.

In previous chapters we introduced the stories of people who confronted very difficult life challenges. In their creative approaches to living, their stories exemplify the qualities of metamorphic resilience — a change and transformation from who they were, to who they are now and who they will become. For example, in Eileen's story in Chapter Three, we hear of disruptions in her education and career, death of spouses, and the challenges of raising a family as a single parent. She is resilient, not just because she met and overcame major life challenges, but also because of her heritage. Inspired by the courageous story of Neengay, Eileen expresses a great determination to overcome hardship and to embrace the future.

Like Eileen, as part of our storytelling we also come to understand our past. Not just our personal history, but the story of our family and community, and others who came before us. From that history, we can gain knowledge of other's struggles, and their story may also serve as an inspiration for us to carry on.

The stories of Meryl and Rick, in Chapter Six, also display the qualities of metamorphic resilience. In their stories we again find manifest the warrior's mindset to continue and fight despite the great challenges and adversities that life presents. Resolute to live independently and authentically, they were excited to explore what their engagement and anticipation of marriage had in store for their future. In their stories we recognize how their creativity

164

and involvement in music aided them to face life's challenges. Their stories, and later in this chapter Rick's "final story," are testaments that also inspire us to continue on as we face challenges in life. Thus, along with Rick's story, we present three more accounts of individuals who we believe exemplify the existential stance of a warrior, living creatively, and authoring their own story.

Jennie Cane

Jennie Cane contracted polio at an early age. This was at a time in the early twentieth century when no vaccine for polio existed. Early in life she was in and out of school, and spent a great deal of time in the hospital. Although paralyzed in the left leg from the hip down and wearing leg-braces, she was determined to have a childhood and life without having her disability get in the way. She was able to study and finish high school. At that time, she wrote an essay on "The Effects of Alcohol on the Human Body" that was submitted in a contest to the Mississippi House of Representatives. The essay won her a 4-year scholarship to the University of Mississippi, and she later completed a degree in law. Although having attained this high achievement, she was also confronted with the prejudice that went along with her gender and disability status. When she was beginning to clerk for her professor, he told her that she was "taking a job away from a man who is the breadwinner of the family." This was at a time where few women held professional jobs or for that matter were admitted to college. Before allowing Jennie to clerk for him, he gave her a physical ability test. He told her to climb the ladder in the library and to bring down a book from one of the upper shelves. Undaunted, Jennie taking on this challenge and pulling herself up by her arms rung by rung—as she was paralyzed in her left leg—climbed the ladder and pulled down the book and gave it to the professor. Later, it was that same professor who wrote her a letter of recommendation to the U.S. Treasury Department in Washington, D.C., to hire her on as an attorney. She would then travel between Washington, D.C., and Denver, Colorado, to work with the mint in Denver. She also worked on RICO cases, criminal and civil cases focusing on racketeering and organized corruption. Her legal expertise focused on logistics and procurement for the military.

She raised four children practically on her own as her husband died in a car accident at an early age. She kept the family together through many financial hardships. One story told by her daughter was that when she had come home during a break from college that Jennie was engaged in tearing down a wall in the living room saying, "here is where we are going to build a fireplace." She also was a great "southern" cook. Growing up in Mississippi, she learned to filet and cook the most amazing, deep-fried catfish, along with homemade hushpuppies and greens. She also was adept at Swedish embroidery and many folks in the community where she lived have products of her handiwork.

She would never turn anyone away from her door, often inviting workers who were working on the roads or powerlines outside the house to come in for coffee and cake. In a display of true charity, she would often say that no matter who they were, she would never turn anyone away who was in need—and she never did. She also related that when her husband was alive that they would be visited by Dwight and Mamie Eisenhower. The former President, who liked to fish, would be taken by her husband, a local fishing guide, to the best spots with the Secret Service agents in tow.

Her story highlights her resilient character and how gender and disability were used as norms to exclude certain people from achieving their goals and limiting their expectations of what was possible. It is still happening today. It takes a truly remarkable person, which she was, not to let the roadblocks of injustice and prejudice stand in the way of her dreams. She rewrites her story through sheer determination not to let anything or anyone get in the way of realizing her goals.[6]

Rick Belcher

We presented part of Rick Belcher's story in an earlier chapter, and we continue his story here. In a way it is his final chapter. Rick Belcher was a self-taught pianist, historian of rhythm and blues, and a rock and roll singer who grew up living with his parents and siblings in Arkansas. He was residing in St. Louis, Missouri when

166

contacted for a series of interviews for this book. As we noted previously, Rick was born blind, and over the course of his life had to meet and overcome many challenges. Nevertheless, he once remarked that he was proud to be part of the blind community. Throughout our conversations he always expressed a practical wisdom about life, made known his great and enduring love for his wife who died in 1999, and his determination to standup for and come to the aid of others, even go to battle to help those he felt have been wronged. During our regular telephone interviews, we also recorded what has become known as "The Telephone Album," a collection of songs Rick performed on keyboard, that also included the rough recording fuzz and sound distortions reminiscent of the early blues recordings of the 1920s and 1930s. The interviewing author first met Rick while visiting his 101-year-old grandmother in a nursing home in 2008, when Rick arrived to give a concert for the nursing home residents. At that time Rick was performing with Professor Mitch Wadley, who as an act billed themselves as the "St. Louis Funk Brothers." Rick started on the piano early in life, but his later stage-performances included impromptu gigs at "BB's Blues, Jazz & Soups" in St. Louis in the late 1990s. A lover of rhythm and blues style, Rick once shared that "rock-and-roll is my religion!" Playing in honky-tonk and Delta Blues style, Rick performed his versions of songs like "I've Got Ramblin' on My Mind" by Robert Johnson, and "I Used to Love Her But It's All Over Now" by Albert Von Tilzen and Lew Brown. Always planning and artistically involved in life, he loved to perform for an audience. For Rick, being a musician was a way of celebrating life and leaving a legacy. Embracing the warrior mindset, he was a person who would walk and stand alone to further a good cause and be a benefit to others. Throughout his early development Rick was aided by loving parents and siblings. He lived with his family until his 40s, when he was assisted by an independent living training program sponsored by the World Services for the Blind in Little Rock, Arkansas. Receiving assertiveness training and other personal counselling, Rick was able to become more self-sufficient and live on his own. With his newly found independence, he continued a metamorphosis of personal growth and self-actualization. In one of our discussions, Rick was asked what he wanted people to remember about him as a musician, to which he poignantly replied:

> Well, what I would like people to remember about me, and I am not necessarily talking about as a musician—I am in a way, and in a way, I am not. As I told one of my sisters, I don't want people to remember me as "that blind boy who lived with his mom and dad"... I want people to remember [me] as a guy who had enough balls to get out of Arkansas—to leave his family, and to go out there to pursue other things and create a life for himself and have his own legacy. That's how I want to be remembered. And as a musician I want to be remembered as somebody who loved music, and loved to rock, and loved to play the blues, and who is happy at what he is doing... and that is one of the best ways you can do it.[7]

Rick's words inform us about life's challenges, the legacy we leave and will write about in the final chapters of our lives. Sadly, Rick passed away during the writing of this book while on vacation in Las Vegas. Rick's legacy and his story is that of a warrior. His life was one of great love and caring for others, and for music. His fearlessness is epitomized in the life he lived and the songs he sang.

Jon Juckem

It is always a great honor and gift to meet a personal hero and to be inspired by their courage. One of the authors had the distinct privilege of meeting such a person one day in his college class. That student was Jon Juckem. Jon's story is quite exceptional. At 12 years of age, he was diagnosed with a cancerous and life-threatening brain tumor. In his early 20s, he underwent a series of surgeries and chemotherapy to remove the tumor, and subsequently additional surgeries to stop seizures that began after his treatment. An outgoing student, Jon was always ready with a comical remark or take on life, and would often stop by and chat at the end of class to discuss lecture topics and share about everyday happenings. He would also mention his health challenges. To hear a younger person discuss undergoing treatment for brain cancer causes one to rethink what is important in our lives. In the many discussions and meetings with Jon, it was easy to realize he had great faith and love for his family, and a special appreciation for people. But with cancer, what chances do you have of surviving to midlife, or even older age?[8] Jon, however, was always up-beat and his resilient attitude inspiring. Throughout all his medical treatments, Jon continued with his education and graduated with a business management degree. He later found employment with a state agency, married, and started his own family. At age 34, Jon champions the understanding that each of our lives, however difficult and uncertain, have a purpose and meaning. Jon's story is one of resiliency and overcoming, and continuing to find joy and celebration in living. As Jon reports, "God gave me another chance for a reason." Continuing to live purposefully, in sharing his story Jon hopes to assist and aid others, saying, "If I can help kids who are going through treatment now or connect with their families, I want to give back."[9]

Marianne Madey

Often it is in our own families that we see this metamorphic resilience. My mom related to me when she was in her 80's that "You kids never knew how poor we were when you were growing up. We ate a lot of potato pancakes and spaghetti with tuna." I told her that we never thought of ourselves as being poor, because I liked potato pancakes and spaghetti with tuna, along with the other foods she prepared that would stretch a meager budget. At that time, my dad was a schoolteacher, and, in those days, teachers did not make much money. But I remember that somehow, he and mom always made sure that we had wonderful Christmases with an abundance of presents under the tree, not knowing how they struggled to give us children (of which were eventually five) the best in life.

Early in their marriage, mom convinced dad to leave his job at the steel mill and to go to college using his G.I. bill from his time in the service to become a teacher. She also spent two years at college and took correspondence courses in painting and drawing.

She painted mostly in oils, but also decorated Christmas ornaments and wine bottles. It was commented at one time that there is probably no one in the town where we lived who did not have something that she created.

She was also the teller of the family history. One favorite story I have is where she relates:

> I just finished watching an old movie, *The Jackie Robinson Story*. It reminded me of the time I was visiting my sister Liz and her family in Brooklyn, New York, in the summer, late 1950's. Liz lived on the corner of Franklin Avenue, which was directly across from Ebbetts Field, home of the Brooklyn Dodgers. On game day my niece and I would sit on the sidewalk curb and watch out for the Dodger players. This limo came by and had to stop at the corner. My niece started yelling, "Hey, there's Jackie Robinson", and he waved. My oh my what a thrill... Memories..." (Robinson played for the Dodgers from 1947-1956).[10]

* * *

In her later years, Marianne Madey took to writing "Odes" about her life, family members, and anything that she could think of at the time. The following is one of her Odes:

Ode to My Life

This evening, I came alive
With such joy in my heart.
I contemplated on staying home
From attending Christmas Eve Mass,
I decided to go.
All of my family was there with me,
St. Gregory's came alive
with so much Glory and happiness.
The choir sang with heavenly music.
With tears I participated in the Holy Mass.
Why would I ever think of missing this glorious Celebration?
Thank you, Dear Lord, for giving me that extra push.
I was unwell for a while,
and missed my parish family.
But they greeted me with best wishes for a Merry Christmas.
I shall now have a peaceful night of sleep.
Jesus, Mary, and Joseph, I give you my heart and soul.

Written in December 2019, this Ode was prescient. Mom passed away the following month in January 2020 following a massive stroke.

The Story Continues

Our metamorphosis begins with telling *our* personal story. When we tell our story, we are placing ourselves on the path toward self-realization and new freedoms. We find that we are not alone. We discover that others share similar fears and concerns. This discovery is not only true in our own lives but also when we see the stories of those from history. Together, in living and telling our stories, we find a way out of the past that has held us back, instilled doubt in us, and made us fear the future. As we tell our stories we

171

recognize what we have in common with each other—the shared struggles, failures, joys, and achievements—that inspire us to work together to alleviate each other's burdens and suffering. The process of metamorphic resilience is not a solitary endeavor. It is an ongoing work that requires help and understanding from others. Importantly, we must also come to an understanding and acceptance of who we are. Psychologist Tara Brach encourages us to engage in radical acceptance. Radical acceptance is "clearly recognizing what is happening inside us, and regarding what we see with an open, kind, and loving heart."[11] Thus, we must acquire a clear vision of our motivations and an understanding of our actions. We must stop beating up on ourselves for our failures, faults, and misgivings. Metamorphic resilience then allows us to recognize that these are aspects of our self and learn to change in a loving way. We accept who we are, and with conviction try to change those things that keep us from being the person we are meant to be. We realize these components of our self can also be found in others. Ultimately, our life is a *shared experience!* One that is understood in the sharing of our story, and in hearing the story of others. Metamorphic resilience thus compels us to seek out loving others and those who will nurture our path toward change and our new becoming.

Our stories call out our past—the good and the bad. What makes us resilient is how we confront the stories we do not wish to tell or are afraid or ashamed to tell. The path to metamorphic resilience is to accept the past as part of what we may have been but no longer are. The path also requires us to accept what is presently happening in our lives, and what the future may bring. Metamorphic resilience is how we face our past, present, and future with resolve, hope, and love.

Release from Resilience

How far can we take the story of resilience? As we alluded earlier we cannot define resilience by emphasizing our differences from each other, what we have gained or failed to achieve compared to others, or how society defines success and failure. But how do we move beyond these boundaries? Through adopting the existential stance of the warrior, living creatively, and in authoring our own story, we move past the previous established boundaries of our existence, those that may have portrayed to us a false reflection of who we are and our measure of worth. In fact, this art of resilience frees us from these restrictive parameters, and allows us to creatively embrace the challenges of our lives.

To practice the art of resilience and experience its power of transformation then is to move beyond the boundaries by which society and how we may have personally defined our sense of worth. We know that we are still afraid, worried, and challenged, but we continue, despite these things! These boundaries are no longer mountains that stand in our way or to overcome, but instead we may view them as rubble, a trash heap that we find is no longer worth wasting our time or energy on. This is a realization of our gerotranscendence, where there is an awareness and recognition that we have outgrown the earlier templates of our life. Where we may feel ourselves to be one with nature, experience a spiritual enlightenment, or express a cosmic anticipation as we draw closer to death and life's final moment of transition.[12] To express a metamorphic resilience then is to recognize that our "living" is a boundless process. That there is no endpoint to our becoming. Although we could proudly mark various milestones in our lives as symbols of accomplishment, there is no place, time, or specific example where we can truly say we have done it all. To engage in a metamorphic resilience is to recognize that we are constantly in transition. We accept challenges and setbacks, and work toward resolutions. We love and receive love, and give and get support from others. We are not held back by comparing ourselves to others, rather we understand that our lives are constantly evolving and changing. To be "alive" is to live in a liminal space; a duality of certainty and doubt; the logical and the illogical; bravery and fear; hope and despair. Our goal is to transcend this duality, to embrace life's struggles with the courage of a warrior, to create, and to live our story.

Watching children, it is easy to see they love to play, sing and dance, create things with clay, draw and paint! Thus, in many ways, as Carleton Eldredge Noyes notes, "The child is the first artist."[1] Moreover, as Noyes suggests, as artists we are "impelled to expression," and in our creativity intone a "hymn of the praise of things." A hymn that expresses a joy and wonder that comes from the artist's being "so bound up with art as to partake of its essence." It is this oneness of the artist with their art, this involvement in its core, that allows for our pleasurable "self-expression and the satisfaction of the need."[2] Indeed, to communicate in lines and colors what we have seen and felt; to emphasize key events and experiences that were most important; to share with others our longings and dreams, as well as our apprehensions and deeper thoughts; these are all part of who we are, and how we satisfy an existential need to proclaim our being.

As children our artistic impulses flowed freely. Later in development, however, we may have steered a different tack and set our creative interests and artistic practices aside. Nevertheless, many of us continue to enjoy opportunities to be creative and participate in the arts through attending a concert or play, visiting a museum, etc.. Thus, in midlife and older age we may welcome the opportunity to begin anew or delve deeper as an artist, designer, photographer, musician, or sculptor. Further, we may feel a desire to shape and recontour our living in ways that allows us to continue to grow as a person and express our true selves. As we have suggested in earlier chapters, we can make adjustments as we move along in our life journey — we just have to think creatively. Thus, much like we might do if we were sailing, we can contemplate and find insight into how the winds blow, and "navigate" later life. We can use our imagination to guide us in our journey. Beginning to plot our course, we may re-examine what might be possible in our next steps in life, and accordingly make adjustments. We may realize that we may not be able to sit at the drawing table or in front of the easel for as long as we did at a younger age, but we can still draw and paint, and be inspired by the beauty of the world in which we live. Still, we are mindful that one may experience health, economic, or other types of limitations that influence how we live. However, these limitations need not constrain us from being creative, or from expressing who we are and what we hope to share with others.

Purple Pumpkins and a Path to the Rediscovery of Creative Potential

In 2009, one of the authors attended the Gerontological Society of America's annual meeting in Atlanta, Georgia. The pre-conference address, *The President's Opening Plenary Session,* was by Erik Wahl, an artist and motivational speaker.[3] The title of his talk that day was "The Art of Vision." Accompanied by a background of recorded music by the rock group U2, Erik's presentation included telling his life story as he quickly painted a rather abstract-looking image on a large canvas. While he painted, he related that as a young elementary school student he loved to draw and color. However, he would later make educational and career choices that would lead him away from his art and into the corporate financial world. At a time when Wall Street was setting record highs, market watchers sensed and knew "what goes up, eventually comes down." Thus, following the great increases, stock prices collapsed in the bursting of the Dot.com bubble in the late 1990s. What this meant for Erik was that his corporate career would not endure. As he continued to paint and talk about his life, he mentioned that after losing his job he met with a counselor to figure out what to do next, and the counselor suggested he take up painting again — something he always loved. Yet, he shared that while growing up, he never felt he was a "good enough" artist to do that for a living. He noted one key event in fourth grade, when he endured the painful scrutiny of a teacher as he was joyfully drawing and coloring a pumpkin purple, who remarked: "Pumpkins aren't purple!" Erik alluded that the teacher's criticism that day dashed his sense of self-confidence and made him feel like his art would never be acceptable. That feeling stayed with him as he made decisions later about college and jobs he would take after graduation. Nonetheless, he maintained his interest in art, but never thought that he could become a professional artist. Until he was out of a job and drawing and painting were suggested for their therapeutic benefit. The events Erik described marked his entry onto a new path in life. One that would involve him painting again, telling his story as part of his motivational addresses to corporate groups, and later publishing a book entitled, *Unthink: Rediscover Your Creative Genius*.[4] The message conveyed in Erik's book is that by thinking outside our prescribed ways of problem solving, we can develop a new vision for our life by finding and recognizing alternative paths. In this "thinking outside the box," we unleash our creativity. And, as we do, we are likely to become better in our jobs, in our relationships, and in many other areas of our living. Moreover, much like the audience that day who looked on as Erik painted, and in amazement watched as he turned the canvas 180 degrees to reveal his portrait of Albert Einstein, through our creativity we can discover new ways of how to imagine and experience midlife and older age. Indeed, even now at this very moment, much like we did when we danced and sang and painted in our elementary grade classes, we can discover new possibilities and pursue our greatest potential as we move into and through the second half of the life course.

From a Fancy Stitcher to Painter and From Saul to Paul

Erik Wahl's story is not unique. We often hear of stories filled with plot-twists requiring great personal resiliency and the unfolding of new paths in life. One distinctive example is found in the story of Grandma Moses, born Anna Mary Robertson in 1860.[5] Living on a farm in Eagle Ridge, New York, she was a woman of simple means and enjoyed making hand-sewn and fancy stitching articles for family and friends. But in her late-60s, arthritis began to make needlework too difficult, so she started to paint. Self-trained, and painting what she saw in her "mind's eye" and recollected about growing up, her art reflects the American folk-art style, and celebrates the natural landscapes and traditions of New England country living. Hoping to earn extra money to support her family after her husband died, she offered her paintings for sale at a local drug store. Much to her great surprise, Louis Caldor, an art dealer from New York City, noticed her paintings and purchased all her works at that time. He later helped Grandma Moses exhibit other paintings she created, thus beginning Grandma Moses' journey into the limelight of celebrity and artistic acclaim. Immersed in her creativity and art-making until the end of her life at the age of 101 years, her paintings are exhibited internationally and hang in museums throughout the world. The career of Grandma Moses, from fancy stitcher to painter and regaled celebrity, champions the discovery of new paths in life and what is possible in older age.

Another historical account of new discoveries later in life is found in the biography of Rembrandt van Rij, the great master painter. Hendrik Willem van Loon writing interpretively about the journal kept by his ninth-great grandfather Joannis van Loon, the personal physician and confident of Rembrandt, relates the story of Rembrandt and the experiences of his great-grandfather Joannis.[6] With intimate insight into the daily way of life of the artist, Joannis van Loon describes Rembrandt's creative practice as a way of coping. That is, in both moments of great economic and personal despair, Rembrandt held that any problem in life could be resolved by continuing in his creative work. Thus, even after the great life disruptions of his wife's death in 1642 and personal bankruptcy in 1656, Rembrandt pursued his artistic practice. Much like Erik Wahl did in the aftermath of losing his job, Rembrandt used painting to maintain a balance during life's most difficult times which helped him return to and carry on a more normal order of life. In reflecting on his own understanding of how to paint, Rembrandt noted processes of transformation which offer insight into his growth as an artist. Describing his intuitions into painting much like a religious experience, Rembrandt after many years in front of the canvas recognized that the artist's use of light, line, and combinations of color are intended to reflect a story about life, a process of dynamic change, of metamorphosis, and of conversion. So that in the moment of creation, like a light shining down from heaven on the road to Damascus, Saul becomes Paul.[7] We may not become a master painter like Rembrandt, but like him we can also find novel insight into our art-making — and discover new understanding in our living and become transformed.

Art Making: A Way to Healing, Wellness, and Wholeness

The stories of Erik Wahl, Grandma Moses, and Rembrandt van Rij highlight the utility of painting and drawing as ways to overcome challenges, embrace wellness, and restore balance in our living. Indeed, both in its symbolic expression and how it is perceived by the viewer, art touches our deepest emotions and aspects of self, and is therapeutic.[8] Moreover, in the creative expression and representative meaning that art affords, whether conveyed and interpreted through the lens of cognitive-behavioral, humanistic, psychoanalytic, or spiritual approaches, art-making is a process of transformation, one that directs and moves us onto a path of healing, wellness, and wholeness.[9] It is not surprising then to find that art therapy, regardless of therapeutic approach or medium, is beneficial for the person. For example, in reviews of the art therapy literature by Anita Jensen and Lars Ole Bonde, and by Steven Clift, participation in both clinical art-therapies and non-clinical community participatory art programs effectively enhance mental health and well-being.[10] Further, for older adults, beyond the positive effects that may come from immersion into poetry, literature, singing, dancing and music making, the visual arts may be especially beneficial in helping the individual form supportive relationships and achieve personal empowerment.[11] For example, research by Adelita Cantu and K. Jill Fleuriet who asked older adults about their expectations and experiences in a community-based arts program, found that engagement in painting, drawing and other forms of art-making helped improve their psychosocial and mental well-being, and strengthened their abilities to focus in a way that is suggestive of better brain health.[12] Moreover, some participants suggested that art-making was like taking a vitamin for your entire body, in that it provided a way to stay focused and mentally active, and led one to an experience of peace and wonder.

Enhancing Cognitive Function and Self-Esteem

Painting and other art therapies are also recognized by clinicians to be important tools to use when working with individuals who encounter neurological impairments and dementia. As Berna Huebner describes in the story of her mother Hilda Gorenstein, *I Remember Better When I Paint–Art and Alzheimer's: Opening Doors, Making Connections,* art therapy allows one to communicate a wide range of feelings which help to restore self-esteem and social connections with loved ones and caregivers.[13] Known as Hilgos professionally, Hilda was a talented young person who liked drawing. Pursuing her passion to make art, she attended the Chicago Art Institute, and later became an accomplished artist and sculptor. In later life, as Hilgos encountered the difficulties of Alzheimer's disease, with the assistance of art students who played the roles of informal art therapists, she was once again able to express a wide range of emotions and creative interests through her art, and continued to paint into her 90s. Indeed, reflecting a Cartesian-like expression of "I paint — therefore I am," Hilgos communicated to caregivers that she remembered better when she was painting! Thus, as observed in art therapy programs for memory impairment and other neuropsychological disorders, art-making provides the individual opportunity for cognitive and social stimulation, as well as imaginative engagement.[14]

Taking a closer look at the benefits of art-making for individuals with neurological impairments, research by Rachel Lee and colleagues involved older adults with mild cognitive impairment (MCI) in a structured art therapy program for nine months.[15] In this research participants created art in a variety of ways (e.g., making collages, drawing and scribbling, sculpting with clay), and also went on fieldtrips to view art at local museums. Therapeutic sessions included guided discussion and sharing of feelings about the art. Subsequent neuropsychologic testing at 3-months indicated that in comparison to controls (i.e., participants who did not receive any therapy and continued life as usual), those who received art therapy had significant improvements in list learning and forward digit span retentions, along with overall memory and cognitive function scores. Further, in comparison to controls, the art therapy group's enhancement of memory function was also found to be sustained at a later neuropsychological testing 6-months later. Leading the researchers to suggest that art therapy used with older individuals as they experience mild cognitive impairments may benefit visuospatial abilities, attentional focus, working memory, and executive function.

As we consider the various benefits of art therapy, it is interesting to note that drawing has been widely used as a neurological assessment to distinguish cognitive and perceptual-motor abilities, and an important form of communication and self-expression for individuals with language impairment.[16] Further, while these applications demonstrate other ways we may tap into and utilize our drawing skills, it is suggested that even thinking of "drawing" an object may affect our encoding processes in such a way that the object becomes more memorable. For example, in a study by Jeffrey Wammes and colleagues, young adults were prompted to draw or write words displayed on a computer screen after their presentation. Following this activity, participants were then tested for recognition of the words shown on the screen. Results indicated that the prompt to draw words following their presentation significantly aided recognition memory, compared to the prompt to write the words. Further this effect on memory was observed even if the drawing was planned but not completed, suggesting that in comparison to writing out the words, that both drawing *and* just preparing to draw the words significantly aided memory.[17] Other research by Myra Fernandez and colleagues involving older adults and adults with dementia, report the same advantage of drawing over writing in aiding memory processing.[18] Thus, just as "a picture is worth a thousand words," drawing is suggested to create a rich context that aids both the encoding and retrieval stages of memory. Further, other research involving older individuals with dementia suggests art-making is a pleasurable experience that engages one's attention, and helps to improve neuropsychiatric symptoms, social behavior, and self-esteem.[19]

Especially for individuals who have aphasia following a stroke or other neurological injury that impairs speech, reading, or writing, drawing is not only an important way of expanding neurocognitive processing, but of communicating as well.[20] For example, much like the findings noted by Wammes and Fernandez already mentioned, research by Dana Farias and colleagues reports drawing may also facilitate the retrieval of word information and picture naming for individuals with aphasia.[21] In this research by Farias and colleagues, aphasia patients were asked to name a picture when they first saw the picture presented to them, or as they wrote the name of the picture, or as they drew the picture. Results indicated that in comparison to the name the picture while writing condition, an increase in picture naming occurred while subjects drew the picture. These findings suggest that drawing aids the connective link between perceptual, associative, and structural aspects of the drawn objects, and the related vocabulary information and speech sounds of language. A follow-along functional magnetic resonance imaging (fMRI) study by Farias and colleagues, examining brain activation patterns of aphasic patients while drawing and writing, further showed that in comparison to the naming and writing conditions, drawing produced heightened right hemispheric activation. Moreover, this research suggests drawing expands neurocognitive processing in a way that aids the aphasic patient in picture naming.

Neurological illnesses like Alzheimer's disease and stroke may cause impairments that affect both the capacity to hold the pencil or paintbrush, as well as perceptual and cognitive abilities that change the quality and characteristics of line, space, hue, and contrast of the art being created. Further, for individuals with Lewy Body Dementia, where there is a build-up of the protein alpha synuclein in brain areas involved in memory, movement, and thinking, deleterious shifts in perceptual-cognitive function may produce impairments so severe that the art produced may appear as very primitive and bizarre.[22] This change in perceptual-cognitive function may not only affect one's art-making, but one's motivation to be creative and the emotional content expressed and conveyed within the art. Yet, when functional or motivational deficits limits one's creative expression, a gallery visit still provides opportunity to experience and enjoy art. For example, an observational study involving individuals with dementia, suggested that visiting an art gallery once a week for six weeks produced memory stimulation, as well as obvious enjoyment and engagement.[23] Further, while memory and social effects were not sustained after the program ended, these researchers concluded that the obvious momentary benefits of sensory, intellectual, and social stimulation for people with dementia warranted that the program continue. As one research participant intimated, when we encounter declines in memory and intellectual function, we tend to focus on the things we can't do anymore, and a visit to the art gallery shifts your perception to make you aware that you can still do some things. Similar positive effects were also reported by Hannah Zeilig and colleagues in a review of museum-based programs for people with mild to moderate stage dementia, indicating that art gallery and museum-based interventions helped to improve mood, enjoyment, sense of personhood, subjective well-being, social engagement, as well as memory and verbal fluency.[24] Thus, whether drawing and painting or visiting a gallery, art therapies provide a bridge beyond the various cognitive, perceptual, and psychomotor limitations that accompany dementia and other neurodegenerative disorders, permitting the individual to grasp and to explore new areas of creativity and personal expression.

Just Doodling?

Teacher to student: Are you doodling during the lecture?

Student: No, I'm not *just* doodling! This is the way I take notes—I make art!!

Like other creative expressions, doodling, scribbling, caricature drawing, and cartooning have been ways of telling a story since ancient times.[25] Additionally, from the perspective of lifespan development, it is recognized that by the time we are toddlers we are already imitating the drawing and writing of playmates and caregivers, and often using crayons and paints to draw the world around us.[26] So, while the teacher might have thought that the student was just "playing around" or bored, doodling during a classroom lecture or business meeting can be a very imaginative and constructive process that leads to much deeper intellectual insights and creative expressions. Indeed, the happy and fun feelings that doodling, scribbling, or cartooning seem to generate can also moderate our mood, and provide a positive framing of the world that affects our decision making and how we live.[27] Furthermore, while certainly communicating basic feelings, interests, and concerns, doodling and scribbling may help people manage distractions and thus aid the encoding and recollection of important information, as well as to serve as a therapeutic tool that enhances learning, self-expression, and self-efficacy.[28] For example, research by Deekshita Sundararaman involving high school students who were asked to doodle in a structured (i.e., shading in a pre-arranged doodle sheet) or unstructured (i.e., doodling on a blank page) way while listening to a history lecture that was later followed by a quiz, reported that in comparison to a control condition where subjects were not allowed to doodle, both structured and unstructured doodling conditions were found to significantly enhance quiz scores.[29] Other research involving college students reports that doodling while listening to a boring story improves recognition memory, but not free-recall memory.[30] It should be noted as well, that while other research has shown that drawing words as they are visually presented very reliably aids free-recall, there has not been consistent positive effects of doodling on other aspects or types of remembering.[31] Thus more research on the possible benefits of doodling on memory is needed.

Doodling has also been used in research exploring ego integrity as a tool for self-discovery and personal growth. For example, research by Allan De Guzman and colleagues used doodling along with puni-making (a traditional Filipino art where dried coconut leaves are folded to make a craft and tell a story) as tools to inquire into the ego integrity of older Filipino adults with physical disability. In this research, both the doodling and puni-making were noted as ways to access and aid the reminiscence process, revealing four important activators of ego integrity (i.e., belief in God, family, work, belief in self). Further, the doodles that participants created before and after the puni-making were noted to reflect and describe a *metanoia* or change in ego integrity. This change suggests a greater grounding, certainty, and integration of the activators of ego integrity that may come about through this type of recreational therapy.[32] In a similar way, other research has suggested doodling and drawing can be used as viable tools in journaling and reflective inquiry to aid self-discovery and personal growth.[33] For example, research by Nantia Koulidou and colleagues suggests sketching that expresses personal concerns, experiences, and feelings, especially those that are often difficult to articulate in other ways, offers opportunity for self-realization and empowering new interpretations of one's inner dialogue and ways of being.[34]

In a like manner, research has suggested caricature drawing and cartooning to be effective tools that can liberate the artist from one's inner critic, as well as other internalized stressors and their accompanying psychological tensions and strains. For example, visual artist and arts therapist Beatriz Martinez Barria posits that when experiencing a creative blockage, drawing a caricature of one's inner critic and naming it, helps to restrain its hyper-critical demands and often self-sabotaging messages. The process of caricature drawing thus provides an opportunity for another, more creative inner voice to enter into dialogue with the inner critic, allowing a moderation between these two aspects of self and our creativity to once again flourish.[35] For example, as Barria reports, a client may draw their left and right hands as caricatures of subconscious self-criticism and the therapeutic expressions of one's imagination, thereby promoting dialogue between these opposing entities and thus an exploration into one's self-disparaging judgments and the liberation offered through art.

Hoping to alleviate burnout and the stress of medical training, Theresa Maatman and colleagues asked medical students to draw a cartoon and share about something stressful in medicine.[36] One finding from their research was that nearly 1-in-5 students reported that the cartooning helped them share about the stressful experience they encountered for the first time; with some students reporting that while they generally do not talk about the stressors they experience, they could now because they had an opportunity to do so. Another finding of this research was that students felt that sharing and discussing their cartooning allowed them to tell their story, connect with others who had similar experiences, and to find solace and healing in the process. Thus, leading these investigators to conclude that opportunities to draw about and share difficult experiences may help reduce medical school stress and student burnout.

Other research also suggests the therapeutic benefit of drawing. For example, in a four-week, pretest-posttest laboratory study by Jennifer Drake, college students were asked to consider the saddest event they ever experienced.[37] Then during weeks one through four, participants were instructed to either draw to express or to distract from their feelings about the event. Results suggested that drawing to distract improved mood more than drawing to express feelings. Allied research by Nicole Turturro and Jennifer Drake inquired into the beneficial effects of participants' creative expression using three different task conditions: coloring a design to distract from negative thoughts and feelings, drawing a design to distract, and drawing to express negative thoughts and feelings. Results suggested that all three conditions helped to relieve anxiety, however, subjects in the drawing to distract condition reported higher levels of enjoyment.[38]

Most of us have enjoyed using crayons and a coloring book growing up. Thus, there have been claims that adult coloring books may also produce positive mood and enjoyment, but it probably depends on what type of creative activity you enjoy most. For example, research exploring the effects of coloring on mood and mindfulness by Brien Ashdown and colleagues, where college students colored mandala designs, suggests that coloring can enhance mood and increase relaxation after twenty minutes of coloring, but were not found to produce longer term effects when subjects were asked to color twenty minutes a day for a whole week.[39] Importantly, as Christine Korol and Kimberly Sogge suggest, the benefits of coloring and drawing to enhance well-being may depend most upon the concerns of the individual, the traumatic events they may have endured or continue to experience, and the person-social context in which they currently live.[40]

More on Caricature Drawing: Having Fun and Finding Personal Insight

As many of us remember from elementary grades, with little concern for what the harshest critics may say, freehand drawing can be fun! When we draw what we feel or see in our mind's eye, it is an expression and communication of our most basic feelings, interests and concerns, and the discovery of new ways we might imagine our world. Thus, an interesting and fun activity to try for your next cocktail-party or long family trip in the car is caricature drawing. Like other party novelties and car trip activities, caricature drawing can break the ice at a party or break-up the monotony of a long journey, and tell us a bit about ourselves along the way. All you do is start by drawing a circle, and then make it into a caricature or a cartoon drawing involving people, animals, or things, and then add a thought or dialogue cloud. Much like doodling, in this simple drawing activity we begin to explore our creativity. The main goal is just to have fun! So, you do not need to be an artist to draw a caricature or cartoon—your best drawing is good enough. Engaging in an activity that involves deep reflection and creativity is a powerful educational tool. Thus, as you read now, please feel free to put the book down and draw anything that you want. Here are some basic instructions, modelled after the reflective journal drawing approach of Emma Tokolahi, to get started: [41]

First, find a pencil or pen and a piece of paper. Then begin by drawing a circle on the paper. Next, create a caricature persona (e.g., a portrait like you might find in an editorial cartoon or animation strip) by adding characteristic features that makes the circle into a person, or into an animal, or into some other entity. For example, in creating a caricature of a person, you might add eyes, ears, mouth, hair, eye glasses, a mustache, then a stick-figure like body to further distinguish unique characteristics of the person that you then might dress in a suit and tie, a dress and shawl, a uniform, a ball-cap; or again, to create a caricature of an animal, add eyes, ears, mouth, and position the body that distinguishes unique characteristics in some way (relaxed posture for easy-going or laid-back, ready to pounce for agitated or anxious, disgruntled by having crossed arms, jumping or running to show excitement, etc.); or, turn the circle into some other entity, but one that has a personality, maybe it's a car tire, a ball, or a long tunnel, then add characteristic features to indicate motion or static qualities (e.g., a spinning tire, bouncing ball, swirling tunnel, stuck in place). Next, create a speech bubble and add text that conveys what the caricature persona you created is saying or might be thinking. You have total license to express what you feel — what is funny, deeply philosophical, a comment on our current socio-historic moment, or a reflection of your personal understanding about life.

When one of the authors incorporated these instructions into an assignment for his college class to help students explore novel ways of approaching and considering important life concerns (e.g., coping during the Covid-19 pandemic, stress from school, relationships, career selection, or moral concerns), and then to interpretively write a brief essay about their caricature drawing, students reported a variety of positive outcomes including enhanced mood state, lessened feelings of stress, and an aiding of their personal development.[42] Moreover, some students noted that their caricatures were symbolic of existential concerns and feelings, and that drawing, while being a fun activity, provided a quasi-therapeutic benefit that promoted personal insight:

> "I love being able to create different things through my art. It was also fun to be able to draw something while also creating a story behind the drawing. I felt like parts of myself came out throughout the drawing process." – Isabella M.

> "It was fun to draw... it felt therapeutic, as if I was journaling or processing my day." – Gracie L.

> "After drawing... I discovered that I have a lot of emotions that I am holding inside and that I should learn to start letting them out more safely." – Amber T.

"I drew a businessman who is not in the best mood. He is irritated by something at work. Many little things were bugging him, and he took it out on his employees he was working with at the time. He is expressing anger and frustration. As I drew this person, I was a little annoyed and tired. I've been working on schoolwork for several hours and just want a break. I think I was expressing some of my feelings in my drawing. This drawing was fun for me... it let me relax for a little bit." – Jasmine S.

"Being creative allows me to express emotions I could otherwise not explain... When I started this drawing... I was in a mood to release... This picture represents that scared person after she found out her husband was leaving but refused to let it crush her. It reminds me of the sadness and grief I felt. It also reminds me of how strong and resilient of a person I am." – Trisha L.

Reflecting a lifespan developmental perspective, perhaps Molly B. summed up best what many midlife and older adults might also feel:

"I've always loved coloring and drawing as a child. I love to create things and tell stories with words and pictures, it's a way for me to express myself even in the simplest way. I think as we get older, we lose that, our way of being creative. As we age, we're so consumed with the idea of having it all together or being an adult. We're preoccupied with school, careers, and families, and we forget to find our spark again, or what makes us, us." – Molly B.

Certainly, as these essay excerpts suggest, even in the simplest drawing there is great symbolic expression and a seeing into the deepest aspects of the person.

Brother A. Brian Zampier's Story – An Artist's Celebration of Hope and Love

As Carleton Eldredge Noyes suggests, the artist's work is a hymn that expresses the wonders of creation.[43] Thus, as we consider the joy of creative expression found in doodling, drawing, painting, and other art-making, an exceptional celebration of hope and love is found in the art of Brother A. Brian Zampier. Born in 1955, Brother Brian's art is captivating, playful, filled with joy, and reflective of both spiritual and contemplative approaches in art therapy.[44] He has sketched, painted, sculpted, photographed, and reflected on art since childhood. A member of the Society of Mary (the Marianists), a 200-year-old Catholic religious congregation of Sisters, Brothers, and Priests dedicated to Mary mother of Jesus, Brother Brian is an artist and social media archivist at St. Mary's University in San Antonio, Texas, and formerly an assistant to the Marianist artist, Brother Mel Meyer. Brother Brian's story describes his developments both in the processes of living and as an artist, and offers insight into how art-making may lead us to find hope and joy in our living. Characterizing an openness to finding new discoveries as we make significant changes and adjustments at various transition points in our life, here is his story:[45]

> I grew up in Utica, New York, as an only child. I have a thing called *ABZ Book of Days*, and it is one of the things I have that is about what I am doing as an artist. I have been doing it for quite a few years, I started it in college in the early 1970s. It is a book that I go back to each day of the year and make a mark. That is one of the things I do every day. I find that sort of neat. I like the idea that it is not finished. That it just keeps growing, and that it changes each time I add something to it. It has been a fun thing to do.

Describing his spiritual and contemplative orientation to art and life, Brother Brian continued:

> I do have another thing, too. Way back I used to get the *New Yorker Diary*, and I have a 1991 *New Yorker Diary* that I use

as a sketchbook. And, now I like to revisit it even many years later, and so I have gone back to this book. It is kind of like a therapeutic process. I feel like the process of drawing puts you in the present moment. You know when you are drawing and looking at something, you're drawing a tree, or you're drawing your hand, it puts you in the present moment. Ekhart Tolle has a book called *Practicing the Power of Now,* and I just like what he says about it.[46] He has a quote that is something like "as soon as you honor the present moment, all unhappiness and struggles dissolve, and life begins to flow with joy and ease." And I just sort of like that.

Explaining the method of using a sketchbook both as a way to develop one's drawing skills and as a form of reflective journaling, Brother Brian describes his early educational training and points of life-transition from student to worker, to entry into the joyful and prayerful community of the Marianists:

I met a drawing instructor in college, Sam Patterson, who said it was good to keep a sketch book, and so I thought I would try to take him up on it. When I first started it took me a while to get into the habit of it. I think my second sketchbook lasted for about 5 years, and then eventually, when I decided to get more into it, and I was going at a faster rate, I was doing something every day. At that time, I did more drawing, where I would draw what was around me. I have a series of those books, and it went kind of fast. And then there came a time that I realized how important it was to date the pages. To put a date on the pages to at least have a record of what you did, then you can go back to it.

My training in college was in graphic design. I had classes in drawing, design, and graphic art. Later I worked at GE (General Electric) as a graphic designer. While I was working at GE, I was at home one Saturday and I was going through the Syracuse, New York diocese newspaper, and I saw this ad for the Marianists and their novitiate site in New

York. And I knew that place, it was only 10 miles from where I grew up and lived. I saw the ad and I passed it, and then I went back and looked at it again, and I liked it. From a graphic design point-of-view I thought it was neat. It had a great headline, "Try Selling it All," and a picture of a Volkswagen, and it was like my car! I love the copy writing. It could still be used today. The ad has a Volkswagen on it, and it says "...just substitute a Nissan Sentra for the Beetle." I had a Chevette. The ad also said, "Life is amazing... we all have a path..." So, I filled out the little response card, and a Marianist Brother contacted me. I found out that there was a community nearby, and I got to know them, and I ended up going there on Sundays for Mass. I had this feeling of, "if I don't do this, I think I will regret it."

Characterizing an openness to experience and processes of self-realization discovered as one moves from one time in life to the next, Brother Brian further remarked about his life-transition from training to be an art-therapist, to becoming a helper for the artist Brother Mel Meyer:

It's funny, but it was like my transition after trying art therapy, when I was a helper with Brother Mel. I never dreamed that I would do that. It was the suggestion of another Marianist Brother who said, "maybe Mel could use some help." I didn't really know that he actually had Brothers working for him throughout his career. So, when I approached him, it was interesting. He knew of my work, and he said, "Well we will try it for a month, and if it doesn't work out, we will still be friends!" And it was like, you know, at the end of the month, I thought this is the dream job—I feel like I really like this! And Brother Mel said, "well, I like what you are doing," and indicated he appreciated what I was doing for him.

The whimsical sketchbook drawings and other art pieces created by Brother Brian suggest the influence of other artists, as he noted:

Charles Schultz (*Peanuts* cartoonist) was definitely an influence. I mean, I had a *Peanuts* collection, and as a young person wanted to be a cartoonist for *The New Yorker*.

Long interested in sharing his creativity with others, Brother Brian has exhibited his work in various art galleries, and shared his approach to art-making in a series of Sketchbook Workshops. In leading a Sketchbook Workshop, Brother Brian encourages each person to feel free, to find recreation and joy in their drawing, and to allow their sketch work to be a pathway to self-discovery. As Brother Brian stated:

> I hope each person will not be afraid, and to make their mark as an artist. To be able just to do it. To take advantage of what you have around you. That is what Brother Mel did so much. He found art. People would give him metal scraps and give him things, and he would turn it into a sculpture, and I was inspired by that from him.

Brother Brian suggests four principles for pursuing one's creativity in any media: 1) Play! 2) Have fun! 3) Do not be afraid! 4) Suspend judgment! Much like the arts therapist Natalie Rogers humanistic approach, Brother Brian shares that he hopes students will be creatively inspired and unencumbered in their Sketchbook Workshop experience:

> What I tell people is that it's important to suspend judgement when you do something. Not to say, this is "good" or this is "bad." But just to say, "well, this is the way it is—I did this, at this time, and this is the way it came out." The more you do the better you get. So, keep plugging away, and enjoy it. I think that it is good to spread joy there, that that's life. You know that there is something there. I need that awareness of the pregnant moment thing, when you are concentrating on doing something, or just like when you are playing music, like the time goes by, and the time

flies with the music and time doesn't seem to even exist. And before you know it an hour has gone by.

Again, suggesting how drawing and doodling in a sketchbook can aid the development of drawing skills and take on qualities of a reflective journal, Brother Brian noted:

> I think sketchbooks can teach you a technique. To have a record of your time to go back and look at, to have… like in my sketchbooks, I have drawings of my parents and their house… and to think that… I know of those lives and when they were alive… and I captured them, at that moment. I think it is sort of a neat feeling because it can bring back a memory. Of a certain place in time, where you were there, and I think it is neat.

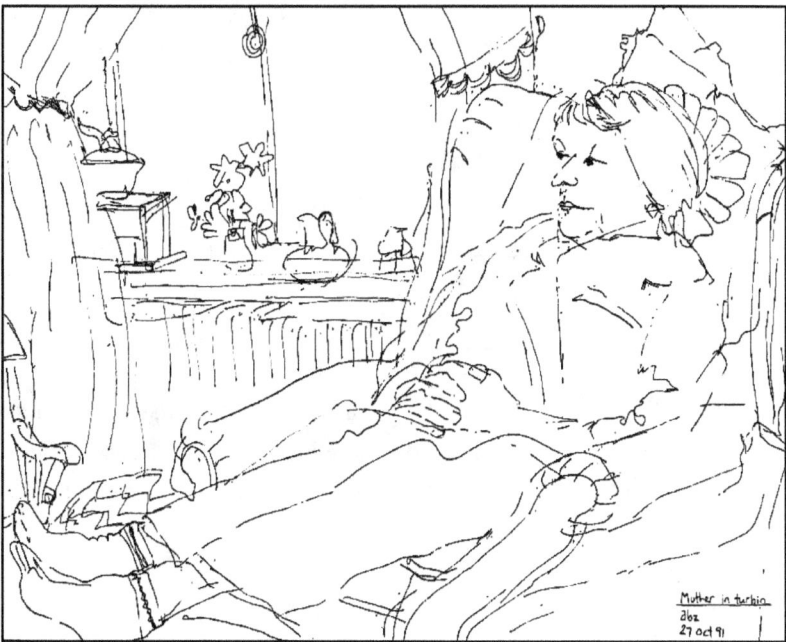

Figure 10.1: "*Today would be her 96th birthday. This drawing brings back memories of our living room in Barneveld, NY.*" *From ABZ Book of Days (https://abrianzamp.wordpress.com/). Used with the permission of the artist.*

For both the young and older artist, Brother Brian advocates the following:

> That they have their own creativity, and you have to inspire them and tell them that it is okay to do it. To try it, and to make mistakes. You know for kids... they love to draw... so then to tell older people that they can do it too!

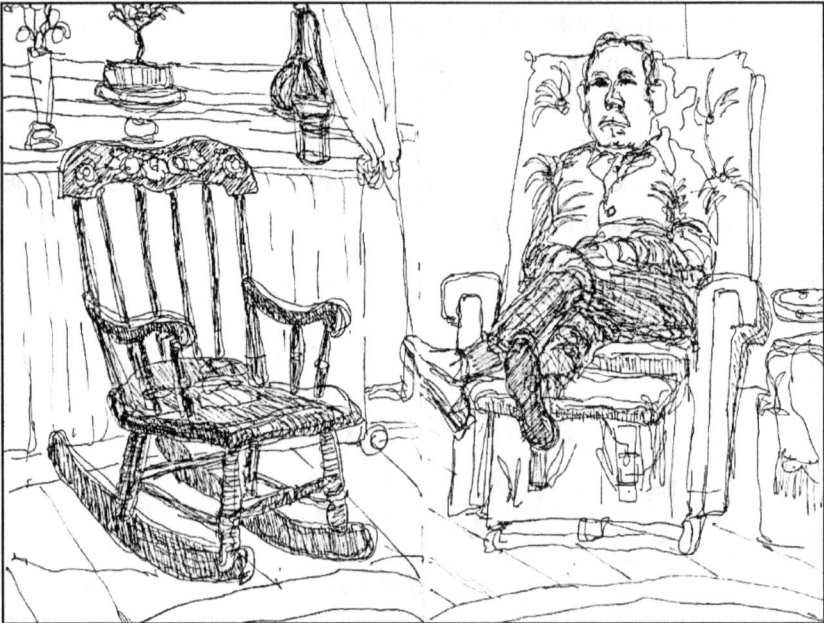

Figure 10.2. *"... a children's rocking chair my mother used... the La-Z-Boy rocker with my Father in it." From ABZ Book of Days (https://abrianzamp.wordpress.com/). Used with the permission of the artist.*

Regardless of whether you use crayons, pencils, or pens, Brother Brian noted:

> There are many interesting things you can do with drawing. You can have people draw with their non-dominant hand, and that can bring back memories. I like to do this thing with kids — I call it imagination drawing; where they are

drawing a square, and then start a line drawing in the square. Like, the line is taking a walk. Just start drawing, and you keep going from one thing to another, and it reminds you of something. And then you keep drawing. Then draw another line and start again. And then when you see all these overlapping lines and shapes, then you can start coloring in the shapes. It's like making your own coloring book, and it is more personal in that way.

Describing more about his spiritual and contemplative approach to art-making, and other artists who have influenced him, Brother Brian shared:

> I got another quote that I really love: "Stop demanding little things." I wrote that in my sketchbook and said, "Etch that on your brain!" And, I have two other people who have influenced me. Fredrick Frank (artist and sculptor and author of 30 books on Buddhism), he wrote *Art as a Way: A Return to the Spiritual Roots*, and *The Zen of Seeing: Seeing-Drawing as Meditation*.[47] Both are about drawing and meditation. He was an artist that went to the Second Vatican Council, and made drawings of the meeting. Another guy I love is Franklin McMahon. He was an artist correspondent, and he would go to presidential debates. He would draw at all sorts of events across the country, and he was at the Second Vatican Council as well. I think that the thing about drawing and meditation, and the thing about Mary's and Ekhart Tolle's always saying "yes" to now, is the acceptance of what is. The acceptance of life as it is. When you are not living in the now is when stress develops. It [drawing and meditation] is like saying "yes" to now. Ekhart Tolle has another quote, "When struggling with the now, tell me what problems you have at this moment." It is like, so there are no problems. Like all the eternal. And, you know, people would ask Brother Mel about his life, and I can remember him saying that, "It was heaven on earth!" That

he was able to create, and do what he loved, and do something he totally enjoyed.

Continuing to be joyfully involved in his art, Brother Brian has taken an interest in the fiber arts, and recently received recognition for his needle felting in the *Annual Juried Issue of the Letter Arts Review*.[48] He has also become involved in the Japanese art of origami. Reflecting on his art-making after the death of Brother Mel Meyer, Brother Brian suggests that both needle felting and the paper folding art of origami are relaxing and meditative:

> Talking about the fiber, you know the needle felting, I discovered that after Brother Mel, when I was on sabbatical. I was in Colorado Springs in an art gallery, and I saw this little sheep, and this little sheep was so cool, and it was made out of wool. There were a couple of ladies there that were fiber artists, and so I went to them and I asked, "what is this?," and they said "oh, that is needle felting." So, I had no idea what it was, until I discovered that you do it by poking. You have this really sharp needle and it has barbs on it. And then you take wool, and the fibers from the wool when you poke it makes it come together. That's how you can sculpt with it. And so, it was like an answer to a creativity problem I was facing. Because with Brother Mel's passing I lost the plasma-cutter (welding tool). I didn't have the plasma-cutter and painting things anymore. Then this sculpting seemed so simple. You could buy the wool roving and turn it into wonderful colors. All you need is a needle. The wool roving is like the raw material you use for spinning. It is almost like cotton candy. You can roll it together in a ball, and then as you start hooking it the fibers come together tighter. It almost becomes like Velcro. You can make different parts, and you can make arms and legs, and then you poke them together and hook them together.

Involved in the Japanese art of origami, Brother Brian is currently conducting the *ABZ Cranes Project* to promote world peace.[49] His

196

plan for this humanitarian project is to give away an origami crane each day, as a prayerful and symbolic gesture to convey a wish for peace. The tradition of making paper cranes follows that of Sadako Sasaki, a young Japanese girl who as a two-year old survived the atomic bombing of Hiroshima in 1945.[50] Living just one mile from ground zero, Sadako was severely radiated. She was later hospitalized in 1954 with leukemia caused by her earlier radiation exposure. During her hospitalization and until she died a year later, Sadako folded cranes each day in the hope of making her wish of world peace come true. Her story of grace and courage as she confronted this progressive malignant disease, and her inspiration to fold cranes and to work for world peace are remembered throughout Japan and the world. Brother Brian also notes the intention of his crane project is to remind everyone of the need for love and world peace, and to convey the hope that we would stop wasting our resources on wars, fighting, and gun violence. Thus, Brother Brian's playful, open, and nonjudgmental approach to art-making suggests an opportunity to find and discover a deeper understanding of ourselves, other people, and the world we share together. Indeed, powerfully reflecting spiritual and contemplative approaches in his art-making, Brother Brian's "hymn of the praise of things" very resoundingly celebrates hope and love!

ELEVEN — RENAISSANCE

In a series of intergenerational discussions involving older adults and college students, one author observed that throughout their exchanges most of the older adults sought to share their wisdom and "best practices" for living. At one meeting, an older gentleman in his 70s mentioned his stern and reactive father, long deceased, and the challenges that arise when one parent never seems happy or satisfied with what their children may be doing. Enjoying a financially well-endowed retirement, he also discussed how easy it was to find steady employment after he graduated college in the 1960s. He noted that he had a sense of job security that he felt was less available for college graduates now. Referring to his failed attempts at married life, he also suggested not to ask him about how intimate relationships work best. Yet, he went on to say that at midlife he found personal meaning in living a religious-spiritual life, and how he hoped to continue to provide emotional support and practical aid to his children and grandchildren—leaving a legacy of sharing, kindness, and love. Incidentally too, he alluded to his recent treatment for cancer and the uncertainty ill-health brings, and how in telephone conversations with an older brother, despite the difficulties with his father, remarked how he missed the "old man." In a sense, he was describing the milestone events and experiences that shaped his development. Moreover, in his sharing he provides us insights into the emerging understandings and new ways of living that might be realized in later adulthood. In this chapter we again consider the arts and artistic ways of living, as well as evolving interests and new understandings found in middle and later life. We will also propose that later life is more than just a period in which we may retire and step away from work and other community involvements, but rather as a time of personal renaissance. A time where one may rekindle earlier interests, reimagine what is possible, and explore novel enterprises as they express one's own unique way to live.

The Second Half of Life: A Time of Personal Renaissance

The French word, *Renaissance*, means "rebirth" or to be born again, to re-emerge. It also denotes a period of Western cultural history, from the 14th to 17th century, in which Europe emerges from the Middle Ages in a revival of the Classical approach to learning, along with great advancement in the sciences and philosophy. Further, during this sociocultural historic period people began to characterize the development of the individual in a more secular way. For example, William Shakespeare through his character Jacques in the play *As You Like It*, written and performed around 1598-1600, announces the seven ages of "man" as they correspond to a person's physical changes and psychological capacities. This monologue starts with the famous statement, "All the world's a stage and all the men and women merely players." The Bard then describes the seven "ages" of our lives. The first age is the infant, "mewling and puking in the nurse's arms." Next comes the second age of the schoolboy, "unwilling to go to school." The third age is the lover, "sighing like a furnace, with a woeful ballad made to his mistress' eyebrow." Then the soldier, "jealous in honour, sudden and quick in quarrel." The fifth age is one of justice, "full of wise saws and modern instances." The sixth age is marked by a transition ("a shift"), where aging begins to take on a more prominent aspect of life. The body changes, and the voice no longer robust begins to take on the "childish treble, pipes and whistles…" And finally, the seventh age, "that ends this strange eventful history." Here we see the advent of the common popularization of getting older as a second childhood, but according to Shakespeare it is a "childishness" that is "a mere oblivion, sans teeth, sans eyes, sans taste, sans everything."

In more recent times, rather similar depictions of the life cycle have been portrayed in models of human development, again utilizing a similar chronology and anchoring periods of childhood, adulthood, and older age.[1] However, in his *A Fresh Map of Life*, Peter Laslett puts forth a new era for later life, a "Third Age."[2] The term "Third Age," is also a concept that originates from the French *(Les Universités du Troisième Age)*, coming about as it was recognized that for many older people, intellectual and physical vitality may continue to be enjoyed well into later life. As Laslett's model designates, the First Age of development occurs during childhood and adolescence. This is a time when the individual is physically growing and involved in efforts to become socialized and educated, yet still immature in many ways and dependent on caregivers. The next era of development, the Second Age, occurs during young and middle adulthood. This is a time when the individual begins to operate relatively independently, expresses greater maturity and responsibility, and can earn and save money. However, the peak at which one may express and realize their greatest achievements and contributions comes later in life, during a Third Age, at the end of one's career and beginning of retirement. The Third Age is a time much like earlier eras of development, in that one may still enjoy relatively good health and be involved in creative, intellectual, and social activities that bring personal fulfillment. Thus, in our 60s and beyond, given that we enjoy good health, we may yet find and experience life's greatest fulfillments. Moreover, much like Robert Browning's poetic expression in "Rabbi ben Ezra," "Grow old along with me! The best is yet to be," in his model Laslett seeks to eschew "maturity" or "old age" as delimiting factors that represent debilities and disabilities.[3] Rather, he advocates that it is in later life when the individual may experience "the crown of life... the time of personal self-realization and fulfillment," as individuals are liberated from child-rearing responsibilities and careers.[4] Yet, this more characteristic "healthy" and active time late in life, is eventually then followed by a Fourth Age. A time much like the older age described by Shakespeare, that of a "second childishness and mere oblivion; sans teeth, sans eyes, sans taste, sans everything." Thus, as also depicted in Laslett's model, the last part of life is described as a time of anxiously wrestling with physical and mental declines that may impede one's functionality and social activities, and that signifies life's ending.

Certainly, life presents challenges for us, and those we confront as we continue into our later years, such as decline in physical health or negative older age stereotypes, will require our best to accommodate and manage.[5] Nevertheless, evidence for a Third Age is born out in the lives of many older adults who continue to work, enjoy good health, and have financial resources that allow them to stay involved in fulfilling personal pursuits and social relationships. Moreover, the stereotypical conceptualization of the Fourth Age, as merely a time of decline and deterioration, has been challenged by Thomas R. Cole in his work, *Old Man Country: My Search for Meaning Among the Elders*.[6] Thus, in contrast to the last era of life being one solely of declines, losses, separations, and increasing travail, Cole suggests there may still be positive and transcendent experiences encountered very late in life that are causes of joy and celebration. Using the metaphor of life as a journey and seeking to regain and augment the humanity of older people in the Fourth Age, Cole suggests that regardless of our age, there is always opportunity for personal growth—always another point of starting again, and composing a new chapter in our story.[7] Thus, in contrast to Laslett's distinction of a Third Age where robust health allows one to still live independently, engaged and fulfilled in life activities, while the later Fourth Age is a time of declining health and functionality that robs the person of self-agency, Cole introduces a reconceptualization of the Fourth Age. That is, that despite the physical and mental declines that may occur late in life, older people may still act freely and live purposefully, finding and expressing a joy for living through their creative expressions, personal meaning making, and social relationships. Thus, borrowing Shakespeare's characterization, Cole adds elements that portray a personal rebirth, where one may experience a "second childishness and mere oblivion..." but also moments of exuberance and fun, powerful feelings wrought forth through experiences in nature or in viewing majestic art, commanding spiritual encounters or philosophical insights, a personal completeness discovered in our family and community relations, and a continuation of and further innovation in our creative expressions or other life-works.[8]

In his research, Cole addresses the existential concerns of uncertainty of being, freedom, belonging, and identity. Examining the stories told by older men, all who held positions of high status and achievement, Cole provides insight into how older age may be a time of continued discovery and renewal, where new meaning and reason for one's life emerge. In their stories, the older men convey the importance of pursuing new creative interests despite changes in physical or mental abilities. Suggesting that through our creative endeavors we can realize a personal renaissance. Wherein we recognize a more profound understanding of the sacredness of each person's life, or a greater elaboration of our spiritual and humanistic beliefs, or find a greater realism in our living and life's purpose. Further, while Cole suggests one may find age-associated decline in libido and physical strength that threaten self-image and identity, there undoubtedly are other difficulties and challenges that shift and redefine one's expression of self-agency. Indeed, there is an evolving expression of personal agency throughout the last half of the life-course. So that, as gerontologists Amanda Gernier and Chris Phillipson point out, even when one suffers cognitive, language, or sensorimotor disabilities, one may express their personhood in the simplest of behaviors and emotional expressions.[9] Even more, as one author realized in sitting with a dear grandmother with dementia, long periods of mental confusion and silence may be interrupted by brief moments of lucid expressions. Moments such as when insightful and humorous descriptions of the social exchange between family members in another room are offered. Thus, as similarly recognized within Indigenous cultures, an elder's personal agency is still intact even when they are understood to be no longer "present" to the community, or as they travel in their journey through the circle-of-life, have "returned to a second childhood," or that despite expressive or receptive aphasia, manifest insight into the supernatural world.[10] Thus, despite one's increasing need for assistance and dependency on caregivers late in life, one is yet a sentient being, and that even through vastly long periods of silence, we may recognize an emergence of new facets and creative aspects of the person.

Metamorphosis and Personal Renaissance

In Chapter Nine, we outlined the concept of metamorphic resilience as involving the existential stance of the warrior, creativity, and life story. It is a process of taking action, of confronting adversity and challenge, and of seeking transformation that adaptively leads to the discovery of new ways of being. Thus, in older age the concept of metamorphosis involves an increasing awareness of one's vulnerability to disease and illness, as well as one's potential to be creative and to pursue personal growth.[11] So that despite physical and mental declines that may come upon us, we may realize new freedoms and possible pathways in our transcendence into the latter moments of the life-course. In continuing in this creative approach to life, we may engage in a personal renaissance and find resolution to existential enquiries posed since our earliest times in development, but still vitally important in later life: How did I come to be like this? How can I be happy? What will the future be like? Therefore, in the middle or later part of the life-course, we may continue a metamorphosis that results in our personal renaissance, where through our creativity we find new hope, meaning, and joy in our living.

Starting Upon the Path of Personal Renaissance: A Poet's Wish

It is through our creativity and self-reflection that we begin to undergo a metamorphosis of being and embark upon a personal renaissance.[12] Our deepest reflective processes are much like an artist's awareness and consideration of color and tone to represent mood, structural forms and movement of line that suggest depth of perspective and transition, contrast between figure and ground and areas of light and shadow that represent points of emphasis, that are metaphors for how we may reflect upon the milestone events of our life, and redraw, extend, or color in parts that have yet to fully emerge. This type of self-reflection utilizes the creativity and imagination that leads us to our personal renaissance.

The insight of those who paint with words, the poet and prose writer, also offers us a model for self-reflection, and the exploring of how we might understand ourselves, others, and the world we live in as we move into middle and later life. Indeed, returning to college to complete a degree in creative writing in her late 50s, Joanne S. Rupp offers us the following concerns and weighing of goals and motives at midlife, that we might also consider as we move toward our personal renaissance:

Relevant Last Wishes

My hourglass is emptying,
Waning, I must prepare,
Waste no sands of time, so few left,
For wishes I have yet unfulfilled,
I wish to be relevant.

I wish to be relevant,
To not be still in my causes,
To share wisdom and mentor greatness,
To be viewed as memorable in just actions,
I wish to be relevant.

I wish to be relevant,
To see beyond complacence,
To defeat obstacles, challenges,
To leave no stone unearthed,
I wish to be relevant.

I wish to be relevant,
To foster creativity, arouse curiosity,
To pursue logical, ethical solutions,
To exemplify positiveness,
I wish to be relevant.

I wish to be relevant,
To light up your day,
To shine as bright as the stars,
I wish to be relevant.

I wish to be relevant,
To show my vulnerability,
To help others realize it is ok,
I wish to be relevant.

I wish to be relevant,
To shower generosity everywhere!
To make life better for others,
After life ends, hope left behind,
I wish to be relevant.

I wish to be relevant,
Upon my last breath, legacy will speak,
Whispers of fulfilled relevance,
Or just mediocrity, time keeps ticking,
I wish to be relevant. [13]

In the poet's repeating phrase to enhance the poem's lyricism, cohesion, and meaning, we find expression of key midlife motives and hopes, and ways to make adjustments to live authentically and to be relevant. Similarly, in sketching out the next steps in our "life-chart" through our drawing, painting, music, poetry, or other creative activities, we begin to fashion a new picture of how we may live, and embark on a personal renaissance where we may strive to be our truest self, and find the deepest meaning and purpose in our living.

Renaissance Actors and Actions

When we play-act, we take on new roles and pretend for a short while to be another person in a different context. Through our theatrical actions and performance, we may sense we have become different in some way. If we played the "hero or heroine" we may have recognized an original power we always possessed, or way to imagine or portray our life in a positive and more effective way. This is another aspect of being involved in a later life renaissance. For example, during one of the author's intergenerational discussions, an impromptu skit writing and role-playing activity was used to break the ice and enrich the exchange between older and younger adults. In one meeting, an especially interesting skit about family dynamics and the challenges of growing-up was at the center of the discussion. The older adults in the skit played the role of younger people, and vice-versa. This brief drama tells the story of a young person, who without asking for his parents' approval, travels to stay with his girlfriend at college for a short time, and the young person's surprise when he finds out that his parents will not permit him to return home. His temporary leave taking had become permanent. While this skit brought up issues of youthful indiscretions, parenting styles, quest for personal autonomy and leaving home, it was also a true story which helped the actor realize a new understanding of this life-transitioning event. Similarly, when we act freely and creatively, in ways that are inspired by our deepest hopes and concerns, we begin to move forward in the process of transformation and renaissance—immersed in a process of becoming and living our own personal truths, where we are no longer just play-acting but rather becoming the central and commanding character of our story.

This freedom to be ourselves, to live our own story, as described by the late Gene Cohen, eminent scholar of the arts and aging, comes from an inner drive that promotes and fosters psychological growth throughout the life cycle.[14] This inner drive manifests itself in the form of a personal re-evaluation at various times in our life. At midlife, in our 40s and 50s, this re-evaluation may be like that of the *Relevant Wishes* voiced in Joanne S. Rupp's poem, where there is concern for the time we have left to live, and the hope to attain lifegoals that have yet to be realized. Thus, as Carl Jung suggested, midlife is a time of shifting focus onto our inner-life, re-balancing intra-psychic needs, and seeking a deeper understanding of the cultural and spiritual antecedents of our psychological "self."[15] Moreover, it is a time of realizing new potentialities and fashioning new roles for ourselves, of reclaiming our powers to be creative, and in reshaping our living so that we may express our true "self."[16]

In our mid-50s to mid-70s, as we again undergo personal re-evaluation we may act freely to become liberated from previous social roles and ways of being. In later life, perhaps greater than at any other time in our development, we have a much broader understanding of our lived experiences and are especially aware of and able to communicate our inmost feelings and inner life.[17] This increased inner-awareness may direct us to a more profound sense of autonomy, feelings of completeness, and elaboration of personal ethics that are now internally centered and individually defined. This new inner-awareness may also release and free aspects of our creative expression and potential for personal growth that have laid dormant. Thus, as Cohen suggests, in this liberation phase, our inner dialogue may be spurred by questions asking, "'If not now, when?,' 'Why not?' and, 'What can they do to me?' "[18] We may also feel less of a need to "filter" our opinions or offer apologies for the life-choices we have made. Consequently, in later life, sensing a new freedom to speak one's mind through our creative expression and in how we live, we may communicate what we feel needs to be expressed, and take on tasks that we feel must be completed. We may also no longer feel a need to play traditional or conforming roles. Thus, unencumbered by earlier roles within family and community, we may live more independently and authentically, fashioning a new life that reflects our deepest truths.

The experiences of later life, however, are complex, and may present other types of challenges. For example, while research suggests an increased interest in positive emotional experiences, and a lowering of neuroticism in expression of personality in later life, there may be declines in extraversion, openness to experience, and conscientiousness that suggest existential challenges in seeing one's life in a meaningful and purposeful way, or feeling "personal growth" is still possible.[19] Indeed, considering the uncertainties that may arise and present further challenge, research suggests that dispositional characteristics, style of coping, social support, health problems, unresolved issues and conflicts from earlier times of development may all impact upon one's well-being, and lead to self-absorption, social isolation, and other negative behaviors in later life.[20] Nevertheless, the liberty to continue to grow and to become our truest self, offers hope that we may experience later life as a time of renaissance—a time of greater freedom of expression and creativity, and of new ways of living!

Renaissance in the Form of Humanitarian Action

Later life may also be a time of greater community involvement and social activism, dynamically propelled by our creative energies, self-assurance, and critical social awareness.[21] In addition, as we expect one's style of moral reasoning to reflect dispositional characteristics, cognitive capacity, and deeply held cultural beliefs, older age may also be a time of moral ripening, where there is increasing ethical and philosophical reflectiveness.[22] Indeed, research on moral reasoning by Simon McNair and colleagues suggests that in comparison to younger adults, older adults are more likely to hold idealistic moral beliefs (e.g., the dignity and welfare of people should be the most important concern in any society), to express negative feelings as they face a moral quandary, and to make deontological judgments (to do no harm to others) rather than utilitarian judgments (doing what is best for the majority).[23] Thus we may sense a new license in later life to take on roles of advocating for others in our community.

Further, we increasingly recognize that the midlife and older artist, musician, or poet does more than just work within their creative media. Through their creative expressions they also play significant roles as cultural interpreters, social justice activists, and advocates for human rights. One example is found in the renowned Canadian First Nations artist Roy Henry Vickers' paintings, carvings, and storytelling.[24] His artwork reflects the ancient myths of the Pacific Coast peoples, and his personal story describes early and later developmental experiences, all of which inform his personal renaissance. It is a renaissance centered in his cultural community, and grounded in the value of each person, the importance of their personal story, and the communal sharing of hope and love. Implicit in is work are the five basic human rights put forth by the *World Council of Indigenous Peoples* at a meeting in Port Alberni, Canada, in 1975: To be free, to belong, to be worthy — just because we are human and part of the human family, to have fun and to seek happiness, and to be loved unconditionally.[25]

An advocate for Indigenous Peoples, social and environmental justice, as well as for those suffering and recovering from addiction, in his personal story Roy Henry Vickers reminds us that we all make a difference in the world. Recognizing the power of sharing one's story, he proclaims, "Storytelling is the ointment of the doctor. The healing salve of the healer... Your personal story makes a difference to everyone that's in your life... [it is] the most important thing you can share with anybody."[26]

When we consider social activism and campaigns for human rights as reflections of a later life renaissance, we find many other examples in the lives of people like Maggie Kuhn, a social activist long interested in human rights. Forced to retire at the mandatory age of 65, Maggie used her executive skills in a creative way to found the "Gray Panthers," and worked the rest of her life fighting ageism and advocating for nursing home reform, elder housing, affordable health care, and the rights of all people to express their sexuality.[27] We also recognize the concern for human rights as a part of one's later life renaissance in the story of Leo Frigo, who after a successful corporate career with the Frigo Cheese Company, in his retirement worked to help those in the greatest need. As a member of the St. Vincent de Paul Society, Leo worked with parolees as they left prison to find jobs and integrate back into the community. Applying his business savvy, he also founded Paul's Pantry, a community cupboard for those confronting food insecurity in Green Bay, Wisconsin. Visiting local grocery stores to ask for unsaleable food, and at times retrieving food from refuse bins, Leo was often noted to say: "It's better that I go into the dumpster rather than making the poor go there, at the end of the day my dignity will be intact and so will theirs."[28] Leo continued his humanitarian work until his death, preceded by and resulting from a fall he took as he delivered groceries to those in need.

In an earlier chapter we asked whom we might consider as a later life role model. It is in Roy Henry Vickers, Maggie Kuhn, and Leo Frigo that we find such people. Others we may aspire to be more like include the environmentalist Bill McKibben, esteemed scholar and founder of Third Act, an organization that encourages people over the age of 60 to come together to combat climate change and ensure our democracy. Awarded the *Gandhi Peace Award* by the group Promoting Enduring Peace, an American peace advocacy organization, and the *Right Livelihood Prize* by the Swedish Parliament, as well as honorary degrees from many colleges and universities for his scholarship and work as an environmentalist, Bill McKibben creatively suggests there is much for us to do in later life. Identifying his baby-boom generation's "first act" to be in promoting and leading the dramatic sociocultural changes of the 1960's and 1970's, and their "second act" of becoming voracious consumers, Bill McKibben hopes that for a "third act," his generation, now older adults, will through sharing their time and money, leave a legacy to future generations of a planet that may still be inhabitable and a democracy that will continue to acclaim and ensure the rights of all people.[29]

We also find role models in Suzuki Yuichi and the Toy Repairmen of Japan, who repair broken toys found all over Japan, hoping to breathe new life into these special playthings loved by children, and bring happiness to all.[30] Practicing the Japanese philosophy of *mottainai*, which seeks to reduce environmental waste and values cherishing the things we have through reuse and recycling, the Toy Repairmen come from many backgrounds but share the same interest in leaving a legacy of caring for one another and for the future. Most of the Toy Repairmen are retired, but all are volunteers. With stethoscopes and screwdrivers, they carefully diagnose and repair the toys that children bring to them. The intergenerational exchange offered by the Toy Repairmen models and celebrates problem-solving, and teaches caring for each other, the environment, and the future. Further, the repairing and restoring of toys practices the zero-waste life approach to living.[31] A very gratifying benefit or "prize" for the Toy Repairmen are the notes and cards from children thanking them for restoring their toy. As Suzuki suggested, a child's joy in having their toy restored also brings him joy, inspiring him to continue to share his time with the children, and to carry on when working on the most difficult to repair toys.[32] Certainly, the later life work of Bill McKibben and Third Act, and Suzuki Yuichi and the Toy Repairmen of Japan suggest ways we may leave a legacy, and continue to write the stories in the later chapters of our life that contribute to our renaissance!

Multimedia Connections and Renaissance in Full-Bloom

There is no greater example of lifelong creativity than Gordon Parks.[33] With keen awareness of the human condition, throughout his career he masterfully captured and told of the life stories he observed through his photography, painting, poetry, writing, musical composition, and filmmaking. Using the camera as a weapon to fight poverty and racism throughout his life, his photographs and films document the ubiquitous and long history of racial discrimination, segregation, economic inequities, and social oppression experienced by African Americans.[34] Growing up poor and in a segregated and unequal society, Gordon Parks began his artistic career as a musician, playing piano in a jazz band and recording his first musical work, "No Love," in 1930.[35] But he soon became interested in photography, as he recognized the camera as a tool to work for social justice. Reflecting his renaissance orientation, throughout his life he would compose musical works that included sonatas, movie soundtracks, and orchestral pieces. A self-taught photographer he would also author the books, *Flash Photography*, and *Camera Portraits: Techniques and Principles of Documentary Portraiture* on technical aspects of photography.[36] Unquestionably, Gordon Parks is one of the greatest and most celebrated photojournalist and glamour photographers of the twentieth century. Working for the Farm Security Administration and for *Vogue* and *Life* magazines through the 1940s to 1970s, his photographic essays are held and prominently displayed by the National Gallery of Art, as well as by other esteemed collections, and known throughout the world. Gordon is also recognized as the first African American filmmaker. He wrote and directed documentary films such as *Diary of a Harlem Family* (1968), as well as Hollywood films such as *Shaft* (1971) and *Lead Belly* (1974) that featured black characters and communities for the first time as protagonists and central subjects of the story, and that introduced to the public the sounds of soul and funk styles of music in the soundtracks. Like his photography, his screenplays and films received great acclaim, with *The Learning Tree* (1968) being one of the first 25 films recognized by the Library of Congress to be preserved in the *National Film Registry* for all time. He continued in all of his artistic endeavors into his 90s, offering works such as the biographic book *Half Past Autumn: A Retrospective*, accompanied by the similarly name documentary film, *Half Past Autumn: The Life and Works of Gordon Parks*, and a final book of photos, poems and reflections, *Eyes with Winged Thoughts: Poems and Photographs*.[37] Recipient of countless awards and honors, including *The National Medal of the Arts*, *The Spingarn Medal* from the National Association for the Advancement of Colored People (NAACP), an *Emmy* for best documentary film (*Diary of a Harlem Family*), the *Living Legend Award* of the Library of Congress, as well as *The Congress of Racial Equality Lifetime Achievement Award*, and induction into the International Photography Hall of Fame and Museum, in Gordon Parks' career we certainly recognize a lifetime of great creative and artistic achievement, celebrating social justice concerns. Directed by Gordon's genius, people discover in his art the humanity we share, and the social justice and empathic concerns that surround racial prejudice, and the inequalities and inequities that racism foments. His life-long work in the arts inspires all generations to pursue a personal renaissance where they may see others as they see themselves, and to champion and pursue societal reforms so that each person may live freely, with dignity and respect.

Technology and Social Media Tools in Our Renaissance

Technology and social media can be used to spur our creativeness—and the associated discovery of new paths of personal discovery and ideas about life meaning and purpose that may arise in the process. We presented in an earlier chapter the challenges musicians faced to stay motivated and to remain in contact with fellow musicians, the audience, and their music during the Covid-19 pandemic. Although they experienced a sense of loss and anxiety about the future of music, many found new ways to stay in contact with and collaborate with fellow musicians. Social media provides a way to create new collaborations with other musicians, to involve a wider audience, and to learn how to use new and existing technologies more fully. As one author notes about his use of a variety of technologies: "I found the shutdown allowed me time to learn more completely digital recording, how to present videos on social media, and to become more focused in my practicing and performing." Further, for almost every form of creative expression and activity, one can find online instructional programs, technology tools, interactive social communities, and attentive audiences. Thus, technology and social media tools may spur our creativity—and our renaissance!

Anyone can become involved in a creative project such as drawing, painting, acting, writing, singing, or by supporting these projects as technical crew, audience, or sponsor. We may embark on a personal renaissance as we focus on having fun and seeing what develops, and suspending critical judgements about whether our own or other's creative work reflects greater or lesser talents or skills. In that way, we create a space to work and perform freely, to practice and to learn, regardless of age. We all get better through practice—and as our understanding and skill set evolves, we can discover new moments in our creativity and a renaissance in our development. Indeed, as we continue into the latter half of life, we echo the words of Robert Browning, proclaiming that the "best is yet to be!"

Twelve — Epilogue: Tell Me That Story Again!

One cold January afternoon, two sisters living in sunny Florida telephoned and asked, "Will you tell us that story again—the one about when you took the dog out one evening and became locked out of the house in the middle of a snowstorm?" They waited for the author's reply with gleeful anticipation. "Of course!," was the response. What followed was a retelling of that story, with added new realizations and humorous insights. In the retelling, there was affirmation of the care and protection we need and offer to one another, even to our pets, and what may have happened if we could not find refuge from the storm. Like many stories too, it expressed feelings, understandings, and hopes for the future. Additionally, being asked to retell the story again is an example of how we are embraced and welcomed to creatively describe and celebrate all the moments of our living with others— even when we are laughably portrayed in a comedic tale. Indeed, as the great humanist and poet Walt Whitman pens in "Youth, Day, Old Age and Night," there is much for us to discover, understand, and celebrate about our lives.[1] And, like the rhythms of day and night, there is a richness and a deepening of meaning and human experience revealed in our later life reflections. Certainly then, as we travel to the end of the life-course and find opportunities to reminisce and tell our stories, we may revel in the grace, force, and fascination of both our youth and our older age. In this final chapter we present our closing thoughts on transcending into and through the second half of life.

Traveling on the Path of Self-Discovery

In a final assignment for a college course taught by one of the authors, students are asked to construct their life-review. For many young people, they almost instantly recognize that they have a rather brief history to consider, and have yet to meet or take on the responsibilities their parents and grandparents have shouldered. For older students, however, there is a growing awareness that "experience is the teacher of all things," and that they have changed, acquired knowledge, or have grown in some way by

214

doing, seeing, or feeling life.[2] At midlife too, as we reflect upon the experiences of our life, it seems easier to gain an historic perspective and appreciate where we began, how far we have come, and what next steps we may take as we move forward into later adulthood. Correspondingly, many older adults report personal insights afforded through reflection upon and review of their life history.[3] For example, in an intergenerational discussion about possible later life regrets, one very articulate older man exclaimed that he had probably made more mistakes in life than anyone else. He related that he had the good fortune to go to college in the 1960s, and after graduation joined the U.S. Army so he could pay off his student loans. The decision to enlist was a way to meet financial obligations, but once signed, enlistment contracts offer little flexibility to pursue other jobs or careers. Thus, he was bound to a minimum number of years of active and reserve duty service, as well as the restrictions of military law. After service to his country, he later enrolled in and graduated from law school and became a lawyer. But working as a lawyer was quite a miserable experience for him. So, hoping to find a more suitable job, he decided to become a high school history teacher; and, as he noted, he loved teaching and helping students. Thus, embracing and "owning" any so-called "life-mistakes" that he could account for, he noted, "they all have made me into the person that I am now!" Similarly, as we review the experiences of our lives, we may discover a deeper way of knowing ourselves. Further, as we consider the arc of our lives and look toward the future, we may also become aware of the next great adventures that present themselves to us as we continue to live our lives. As we noted in Chapter Three, however, reminiscing and life-review may not necessarily be free of emotional challenge. But like the story of the soldier-lawyer-high school teacher just described, in talking about our experiences, we continue to learn about life.

The Deeper Psychologies of Later Life

As we find in the stories presented throughout this book, later life is much more than a time of increasing risk for illness, physical or mental declines, social separations, or living in seclusion. As Meryl Shechter with great resilience alluded in Chapter Six, "life teaches you—both your head and your heart... and while there are ups and downs, when you are down you can always get up again." Thus, despite declines and changes that may come upon the person in later life, it is also a time for new adventures, and of new ways seeing the world. It is also a time of finding deeper meaning, greater personal fulfillment, and new ways to contribute to our family and community. Even at the moment of death, there may be new insights expressed and shared. For example, as one colleague related, he sat vigilant at his mother's bedside while she slept and came to the end of her battle with cancer. As that final moment grew closer, she suddenly awoke and turned to her son and said, "now I know," and then she laid back, closed her eyes, and died. This final exclamation of awareness, as Michael Nahm and others also report, shows that even in our very last moments of life, we experience new insights and understandings.[4] Indeed, the many personal transformations we undergo as we move through the life-cycle, from the very earliest times of childhood to the time of death, suggest there are much deeper psychologies to explore and understand as we transcend the life-course. As a result, perhaps it is only at a critical moment during our older age, that we begin to grasp the complexities and begin to gain insight into the deepest meanings of our lives.

One of the foremost paradoxical concerns is how we viewed ourselves in the past, and how we may adaptively see ourselves in the present and in the future. As the ancient wisdom expresses, "We don't see the world as it is, we see the world as *we* are!" This consideration of how our perceptions shape how we think and act is also realized in research that seeks to understand the person in development.[5] Thus, with great bewilderment at times, we may have difficulty seeing beyond our own distortions or subjective reality, and understand our experiences of growing older.[6] Two rather concrete examples of how the way we see the world affects how we act are worth noting: The first comes from the artist Roy Henry Vickers (introduced in Chapter Eleven), who reports he always dreamed of becoming a member of the Royal Canadian Mounted Police.[7] But to do so requires that one can distinguish the different hues of the color-spectrum, and Roy was color-blind. So that dream-career was not possible. Ultimately, however, Roy eventually found his life-calling as an artist. His unique color perception is an integral part of his art and the beautiful paintings he creates. The second example is provided by Victoria Jicha, the musician and fancy stitcher we learned about in Chapter Four. Describing a rather unique ability, Victoria relates, "This is going to sound egotistical, but I believe that some of us are born with special gifts and mine is the ability to hear, and to see what I hear. I have perfect pitch and chromesthesia (where auditory information may be automatically experienced in the visual system so that it evokes an experience of color or shape or movement). Anyway, that gift has provided me with an interesting career."[8] Certainly perfect pitch is a gift all musicians cherish, but the perceptual phenomena of auditory-visual synesthesia provides for a more imaginative and richer way of being involved with music.[9] Thus, like the color-blind artist or musician with chromesthesia, how *we* are shapes and filters how we see the world, and leads us onto the various paths we travel in life. At midlife and in older age too, our earlier life-experiences filter and shape the way we see the processes of aging and getting older, and how we move along in our journey. By being aware of our unique way of seeing the world, and how our perceptions provide the basis for our creative, analytical, and critical thinking, as well as our biases and distortions, we may discover an enriched way of living and renewed connection with the world around us as we continue and move into later adulthood.

Clearly, throughout life we are involved in an adaptive quest to live comfortably, to have positive relationships with others, and ultimately to make our lives meaningful.[10] In later life too, as career and family or social involvements wane, we may seek to overcome the challenges of social exclusion, feelings of personal obsolescence, and the despair we might feel about the difficulties we have faced or the life we have lived. We hope to be resilient as we endure chronic illness or life-threatening disease. Adaptively along the way, many of us come to the realization that life's greatest hardships can also lead to our greatest successes![11] As we have suggested throughout our discussion, our creativity provides us a pathway to confront and overcome the challenges we face in life.

Yet, as we move forward, we also are challenged by the distorted beliefs or entrapments of aging.[12] For example, these entrapments include believing that aging can only be defined in medical or pathological terms, or through dichotomous frameworks such as successful-unsuccessful, healthy-unhealthy, and positive-negative. Further, entrapments of aging include the distorted belief that aging itself is just the depiction of cognitive or physical declines, or that in later life we have little to share with or offer to others. As we consider later life creativity, entrapments of aging may involve thinking that I am not imaginative or cannot be expressive, or that my sketches or paintings are not good enough to share with others, or holding the notion that one has to be better than the other clarinetists in the band, or everyone has to like my wood carvings or poetry. It is these beliefs that continue to stymie and hold us back from experiencing the joys that may be found in our creativity. As expressed in the many personal stories shared throughout this book, we believe later life to be a time of greater awareness, offering us new freedoms and novel opportunities. It is a time when we may create and work to leave a legacy of caring for others and for the environment—offering a bequest of love and compassion, and an approach to living that holds respect for all. Further, we suggest that it is through our creativity and artistic expressions that we leave an inheritance that tells of our lives, our moments of transformation, transcendence, and ultimately becoming who were meant to be. Thus, as the poet, novelist, and critic Theophile Gautier similarly expresses—our creativity is a celebration of one's life and legacy for its own ends.[13]

"Breaking Through (To The Other Side)"

In their debut album, the rock group the Doors sing of "Breaking Through (to The Other Side)." Their song is symbolic of the continuing processes of change, discovery, and new understanding that we experience in the course of our living. Throughout our discussion we have implicitly alluded to moments of breaking in, of breaking out, and of breaking through. These processes of becoming are depicted as various moments in our personal journey of transformation and self-realization.[14] With this allegory in mind,

"Breaking Through" was included by the National Aeronautics Space Administration (NASA) in the playlist that aroused the robot explorer *Curiosity* every morning during its mission to Mars.[15]

Correspondingly, in the stories and research presented here, we find many examples of how the arts of living provide us a new way to "breakthrough" in our becoming and continued development in later life. Ways that through our creativity, as we approach the altar of imagination and encounter the sacred ritual of self-expression, we begin to see reflected in our intra- and interpersonal mirror what is yet possible in life. Indeed, when we listen to songs, watch dramatic programs, become engrossed in a sitcom, or become the sculptor, gardener, musical composer, sketch artist, painter, or poet, we encounter and respond to communal situations and life-questions that portray aspects of our own experiences and concerns. In these creative involvements we become imbued with a nurturance and inspiration that enhances our well-being, and that brings to the forefront the many areas of our lives that are worth celebrating

Throughout our global community we find people of all ages and backgrounds coming together to celebrate their living through the arts. For example, the Houston Methodist Hospital's Center for Performing Arts Medicine (CPAM) directed by J. Todd Frazier, offers a one-of-a-kind health care for performing artists that considers their unique needs, but also recognizes the arts as a key component of the holistic care and life orientation they hope to make available to all their patients as well as members of the broader community.[16] Directed towards realizing the potential for the collaborative integration of the arts and medicine in health care, Houston Methodist's CPAM embraces four comprehensive goals in its undertaking: To provide health care and wellness education for performing artists; to offer meaningful and effective combination of performing and visual arts within the health care environment; to incorporate therapies that integrate and utilize the arts in patient care; and, to research and explore the utility of the arts in the areas of clinical therapy, rehabilitation, and human performance. Thus, nearly every day of the year there is a free lunchtime concert in the Crain Garden of Houston Methodist Hospital, supplemented with approximately 150 other special performances throughout the year.[17] Along with music programs, paintings, photos, drawings, and sculpture are also found in gallery spaces throughout the Houston Methodist system of eight hospitals. This integration of the arts into the health care environment is intended not only to enhance patient comfort and wellness, but also employee, staff, and visitor's well-being.[18]

Research exploring how the arts integration programming of Houston Methodist impacted patients and employees during the Covid-19 pandemic indicated many beneficial results. For example, playing music and voice recordings for medically sedated patients was noted to produce positive stimulation effects, enhancing well-being of patients and support staff.[19] In another application, the innovative use of kazoos to help patients strengthen diaphragm and lung capacity was suggested to improve respiratory function and bring great levity and humanity to the entire health care team during this critical time. In an intervention incorporating passive art experiences, researchers used closed-circuit viewing of a live music concert or of a painter as they painted a picture to provide cognitive stimulation and temporarily transport the patient from the hospital setting into the beauty of a more natural environment. Further, through a printed invitation on the three daily meal trays that patients receive during their stay in the hospital, researchers offered individuals a way to participate in inventive and self-guided reflective art activities such as creative writing, replacing lyrics in songs, the origami art of paper folding, free drawing, or drawing their family crest. These activities were suggested to involve the patient in the reflective process of creating, allowing the individual to delve into and express novel interests, convey key aspects of their personhood, and reflect upon their family, pets, and other supportive relationships. Other arts and music integration programming involving staff and employees was also suggested to promote personal and community resiliency, and provide a sense of hope during the pandemic.

Beyond the beneficial effects noted in health care settings, we also find many local community art experiences that aid and enhance mind-body-spirit wellness. In particular, a trip to any museum is an immersive experience that engages the individual in reflecting upon the imaginative processes that underlie and are found in painting, sculpture, architectural design, and historic artifacts. For example, *Seismique*, an interactive art experience also in the Houston area, allows viewers to enter and explore different dreamworlds, revealed in exhibits containing engaging technology, and surrealistic architecture, art, and design.[20] Similar immersive engagement experiences in nature and its therapeutic benefits may be realized through a visit to a nearby park, nature center, or botanical garden. Moreover, these types of immersions might be as close as your backyard or local public garden. For example, regardless of available backyard space, you might create your own garden, where flora and landscape intersect to create a portal that leads to a deeply reflective and refreshing encounter with nature.[21] As we experience the beauty of the garden and engage all of our senses, we become aware of the long human history of garden design and plant cultivation, the healing power of working the soil, as well as the great personal satisfaction and joy of planting, observing growth, and reaping the harvest.[22] Further, it is noted that as a community activity, gardening brings people together in a way that allows us to cross a bridge that spans generational and cultural differences, and that encourages better nutrition, improved health and well-being, and enhanced vitality in our living![23]

Hands-on involvement in other artistic areas may also serve as a bridge to the other side, where we may discover deeper insight into the meaning and purpose of our lives, as well as opportunities for new involvements and connections with other people. One bridge is New Horizons, a community-based music program found across the U.S., Canada, as well as Internationally. New Horizons provides a pathway for adults of all ages interested in making music, regardless of whether or not they are a "beginner," or have past or current musical experiences. It is a creative involvement where one may improve their musical abilities, meet and make new friends, perform in concerts, and where one may discover firsthand music's vital influence upon and connection to life.[24] Moreover, as suggested by the founder of New Horizons, Dr. Roy Ernst, through listening to and making music, regardless of one's level of sophistication, the power of music becomes transformative and offers a variety of ways for the person to improve one's physical and mental well-being.[25] Other similar community ensembles include drum and bugle corps, and community or adult bands, which also seek to enhance members social experiences and provide opportunities to enjoy the excitement and joy of musical performance.[26] Forming a "garage band," instrumental duet, trio, or small ensemble are also other avenues one may travel to find joy and fulfillment through music making.[27]

For folks who find joy in singing, organizations like Chorus America, The Barbershop Harmony Society, and the International Federation for Choral Music, also offer opportunities to meet other people, engage with diverse communities, and benefit from the enrichment that singing and music offers.[28] As correspondingly found with instrumental ensembles, research suggests involvement in a community singing group significantly reduces feelings of loneliness, and is associated with better mental health, physical vitality, and well-being, as well as improvement in respiratory health and reduced pain intensity. [29]

We do a lot of re-creating ourselves as we move along in our lives. Moreover, in later life, as we look back and look ahead, we might discover new insight. For example, as Victoria Jicha noted in her own personal reflection, "If I Only Knew Then What I Know Now," "in older age we are not able to continue to be the same persons we were in our 20s — and who would want to do that anyway?"[30] As we continue in our journey throughout life, we make many changes and transitions, and in each evolution we come to see a new transformation of ourselves. This transformation requires us to adjust and rethink our approaches to living. In essence, we reimagine what may be possible and how to artistically continue in our living as we grow older. It may mean that we adapt or modify our creative activities in some way as we enter the shadow of mental and physical decline or confront the looming specter of Alzheimer's disease. Thus, another program that offers a pathway as we seek to continue to express ourselves and grow as a person, is the Alzheimer's Poetry Project (APP).[31] Founded by Gary Glazer and providing programming in the U.S., Canada, and

Internationally, APP seeks to continue to recognize the personhood of the older adult with dementia, as well as their ongoing potential to create. Importantly, the APP provides the elder with dementia an outlet for their self-expression through the creation of poetry, and in the process continues to celebrate the elder as a member of the human family, communicating to the individual their value as a person and their ongoing importance in the community. This recognition of the basic need to express oneself and to continue to explore self-growth through the process of creating, is also noted in research that demonstrates the very exceptional painting and drawing of adults with frontotemporal lobe dementia.[32] Thus, adult day-care and other community programs that offer arts-based therapies for those with cognitive impairment are noted to enhance feelings of inclusion and quality-of-life, and assist the elder in their continued self-expression and social communication.[33] They also advocate for continued recognition of the elder as an important member of the community, and their potential for enhanced and emergent artistry, even when neurological illness or injury affects the person's thinking, feeling, and acting.[34]

Throughout the world we see pioneering individuals and forward-looking organizations championing the arts as an integral part of our lives. To grow strong the programs within our communities, some countries offer a variety of arts-based tool kits to use as a way of engaging and bringing communities together.[35] Indeed, throughout the globe, integrative arts, music, and other creative community programs are found to strengthen social networks and make connections between diverse groups, as well as offer involvement in the arts to enhance mental and physical well-being for everyone.[36] Further, it is also through participating in community involvements such as a quilting group, a free painting and art studio, or a book club, as well as contributing one's services to a local habitat for humanity building program, or an elder life story project, or a senior center arts exhibit, or an adult day-care arts initiative, that we find opportunity to assist older adults and recognize them as valuable participants in creating our tapestry of life. It is through understanding, respect, and compassion that we all come to know that we have unique gifts that contribute to a celebration of our living.

Along with these types of community involvements, we may also consider taking up more personalized hands-on activities such as the arts of ceramics, sculpture, or woodworking, or writing about our lives or making audio-visual recordings, as ways to leave a legacy to our family and the generations that follow.[37] In all these creative endeavors we may learn new techniques, explore new areas of self-expression, and develop an historical record that documents the arc of our creativity. For folks who wish to explore and create without the constraint of critical boundaries, perhaps developing a *zine*, a self-published integrated print-work may be something to consider. A zine may include any combination of text and graphic media, and while often personalized, can focus on any topic. Thus, zines may contain dramatic stories, drawings, photographs, poetry, cartooning, or other creative ideas and expressions. Importantly, the main rule in zine making is that there are no rules![38] In a world facing such great challenges as ours, pursuing our creative expressions in zine making is another way to breakthrough, and to begin to convey the hopes and dreams we hold for our families, friends, and community.

Getting Started – Finding Our Way Back to the Garden

It is often noted that the greatest and most treasured gift we give, is one we make with our own hands. Indeed, we cherish the hand-knit socks or caps received at holiday time, find joy in creating home-made birthday cards, and often discover new insight and understanding in the hand-drawn cartoon. We find our place in relation to nature as we toil in the garden and later gather the homegrown crop that we will share with neighbors. As we draw, paint, dance, make music, sing, quilt, and write about our lives, we express and pass on our understanding, wisdom, and hope to our families and others in our community. Moreover, we communicate the excitement, adventure, and joy we find in our living—and in the process break through to the other side, rising to new heights as we are taken up by the spirit of imagination, understanding, compassion, and the wonder that we share. In Chapter Four we suggested that through our creativity we may delve deeper into what makes us who we are, and discover new aspects of how we may be that reflects and leads us back to the source of our being. Where, much like when we visit a lovely garden, we find tremendous beauty and stand in awe of the power that creates and designs worlds such as these. In this garden we find comfort and revitalization as we imagine what is yet possible for us as we continue on into later life. But how do I find my way back to the garden? How might I start?

We may begin to find a path back to the garden by following the guide to creativity suggested by Brother A. Brian Zampier in Chapter Ten: play; have fun; do not be afraid; suspend judgment. Life is more than all the toil and struggles that we encounter on our journey. Regardless of however unhappy our present experiences, or how despairing our future may seem, we may continue to describe moments of hope, and find respite and rejuvenation in our creative works. We are inspired by the efforts of older and younger people who continue to practice their arts of living, sharing their dreams about what may be possible in the middle and later parts of life, and who reflect the awe-inspiring wonder and goodness we may yet discover in the world. They have helped us to consider new ways by which we may refine and express ourselves through various creative activities. They have also helped us break out of old habits and frameworks for thinking that limit the possibilities of how we might live creatively, freely, and happily. With their support we sense a greater force that pushes us to breakthrough and to find deep meaning in our lives. No longer do we need to be held back by the anchor of youth-centered beliefs or stereotypes of what later life might be, or what should be expected in our creative efforts and activities.

As we seek a pathway to joy and fulfillment in later life, perhaps just framing our search in a way that adopts an orientation of playfully experimenting to see what happens, and relieving ourselves of any predetermined ideas about what should be accomplished or how good our efforts might be, will allow us to discover a point of entry into this garden. As noted throughout our discussion, we might find and re-enter this garden again through our trek into natural settings, practicing tai chi or qigong, or in dusting off an old musical instrument and beginning to play at home or with others again. We might visit an art museum or sculpture garden, or gather pens and begin to draw and experiment as we did in elementary school, or enroll in a community arts program, or take more formal classes in painting or ceramics. We can become involved with a community theatre group, as an actor, member of the crew, or in another supporting role. We can blog our poetry, short stories, offer other creative articles in social media, or join and become involved with others in a writing group. There are many creative pathways open to us where we can find new opportunities for self-discovery, joy, and fulfillment in later life. Let your creativity direct you—back to the garden—to the place you have always known and where you find comfort, hope, and love.

Coming to a Happy Ending

In our gerotranscendence, as we encounter and experience age-related illness, physical and psychological declines, and the surrealistic impairments to our living they present, we may feel like our life is relatively over, or what we do or who we are does not matter much anymore.[39] We may become bogged down by ruminations and regrets about our past, or anxieties about the future. We may feel so overwhelmed by the challenges we face, that our very existence seems threatened. Like the very devastating effects of the Covid-19 pandemic described in Chapter Eight, where the magnitude of death and disruption to our way of life was so impactful that many gave up hope of any future beyond the disease, we also saw that after a "dark night of the soul," people could find a balance again in and through their creative expression. And once again move forward, in a celebration of life!

As we proposed in Chapter Nine, it is through the fearless and persevering stance of a warrior, our need to create, and the telling of our stories that we uncover what molds us and defines our human existence. Throughout our discussion we have suggested how our lives are experiential and best lived-in mindful reflection of the current moment. We have also proposed that there are many arts of living — that through various creative activities, crafts, and hobbies, as well as other imaginative pastimes and ways of being, we may discover new insight about ourselves as we continue our path in life. Further, we have suggested that in our creative expression we may leave a legacy that communicates our insights, hopes, and concerns to others as we travel along in our final transition. Nevertheless, as a storyteller of our life we wish not only to relate the ups and downs, the hardships and successes, the despair and triumph of our experience, but also to provide the listener a sense of meaning and a resolution to the story with a happy, or at least hopeful ending — and there is a happy ending for all of us to realize. Indeed, as the great poet Walt Whitman suggests in "Twilight," just as the sun that passes beyond the horizon in the evening, we may offer our creative legacy to others as we tell them of our final moments in our journey, moving forward into the eternal night, and our hope of finding respite, nirvana, oblivion.[40]

Join in the Celebration!

Finally, we like to think that becoming involved in a celebration of the arts of living, is something that will benefit people of all ages and walks of life. We believe each person is more than the sum of their physical limitations or health issues; more than the limits of their economic wherewithal and housing arrangements; more than their humble achievements or special "statuses." We embrace the importance of seeing older people and older age through a lens that seeks to explore the experiential, existential, and continuity aspects of living. We recognize that our creativity, learning, and processes of adaptation do not end as we continue to move to the very end of the life-course. Indeed, perhaps it is in later life that we discover that we have so many more gifts yet to share with others. It is through our unconditional acceptance and compassionate communication that we can send a message to others that their lives and their stories are important and valuable too—just because they are who they are. In the last chapters of our life, as we seek to write and to live out our happy ending, we understand that we will be changed by the processes of aging. Yet, there is always the possibility of new learning, and finding new ways of being. In the telling of the mystery and adventures of our life, in sharing our creative expressions, we join our story to the great tome. Indeed, it is through our celebration of the arts of living that we ultimately discover a path toward joy and fulfillment, and by which we realize our transformation as we confidently transcend midlife, move into older age, and approach the end of our life.

NOTES

PREFACE TO THE CELEBRATION OF THE ARTS OF LIVING

1 Rene Doumic, *George Sand, Some Aspects of Her Life and Writings*, Alys Hallard, trans. (in the public domain, 1910): 304-308.

2 Scott F. Madey and Dean D. VonDras, *Music, Wellness, and Aging: Defining, Directing, and Celebrating Life* (Cambridge University Press, 2021).

3 Natalie Rogers, Keith Tudor, Louise Embleton Tudor, and Keemar Keemar, "Person-Centered Expressive Arts Therapy: A Theoretical Encounter," *Person-Centered & Experiential Psychotherapies 11*, no. 1 (2012), pp. 31–47.

CHAPTER ONE – TOWARDS A CELEBRATION OF THE ARTS OF LIVING

1 Walt Whitman, "To Old Age," *Leaves of Grass* (in the public domain, 1867).

2 Jan Baars, *Aging and the Art of Living* (JHU Press, 2012).

3 Carl Gustav Jung, *Memories, Dreams, Reflections* (Vintage, 1989).

4 See for example the following works: Max F. Fuller, *The Sacred Books of the East* (Oxford at the Clarendon Press, 1882). Ronald J. Mason, *Inconstant Companions: Archaeology and North American Indian Oral Traditions* (University of Alabama Press, 2006). Oswaldo Chinchilla Mazariego, *Art and Myth of the Ancient Maya* (Yale University Press, 2017). John Sawyer, *Sacred Languages and Sacred Texts* (Routledge, 2012). Peter R. Schmidt, *Historical Archaeology in Africa: Representation, Social Memory, and Oral Traditions* (Rowman Altamira, 2006). Gerald P. Verbrugghe, and John Moore Wickersham, *Berossos and Manetho, Introduced and Translated: Native Traditions in Ancient Mesopotamia and Egypt* (University of Michigan Press, 2001). David S. Whitley, *Cave Paintings and the Human Spirit: The Origin of Creativity and Belief* (Prometheus Books, 2009).

5 See for example works by Aristotle, Jonathan Barnes, ed., *The Complete Works of Aristotle*. Vol. 1 and 2 (Princeton, NJ: Princeton University Press, 1984). Wing-Tsit Chan, *The Way of Lao Tzu* (Ravenio Books, 2015). Benjamin Jowlett, *The Complete Works of Plato* (Akasha Publishing, 2008). Charlene Tan, *Confucius* (A&C Black, 2014).

6 C. G. Jung, "The Structure and Dynamics of the Psyche," *Collected Works of C. G. Jung, 8* (Princeton, NJ: Princeton University Press, 1970); Abraham Maslow, *Toward a Psychology of Being* (New York: Simon and Schuster, 2013); Rollo May, *The Courage to Create* (New York: WW Norton & Company, 1994); Rollo May, Ernest Angle, and Henri F. Ellenberger (eds.), *Existence* (New York: Clarion Books, 1958); Carl R. Rogers, *On Becoming a Person* (Boston: Houghton Mifflin Company, 1961); Irvin D. Yalom, *Existential Psychotherapy* (New York: Basic Books, 1980).

[7] Lars Tornstam, *Gerotranscendence: A Developmental Theory of Positive Aging* (New York, NY: Springer Publishing Company, 2005). Lars Tornstam, "Stereotypes of Old People Persist. A Swedish "Facts on Aging Quiz" in a 23-year Comparative Perspective," *International Journal of Ageing and Later Life* 2, no. 1 (2007): 33-59.

[8] See reviews concerning hemispherectomy by the following: J.S. Kim, E.K. Park, K.W. Shim, and D.S. Kim, "Hemispherotomy and Functional Hemispherectomy: Indications and Outcomes," *Journal of Epilepsy Research, 2018 8(1)*, 2018:1-5. E.P. Vining, J.M. Freeman, D.J. Pillas, S. Uematsu, B.S. Carson, J. Brandt, D. Boatman, M.B. Pulsifer, and A. Zuckerberg, "Why Would You Remove Half a Brain? The Outcome of 58 Children after Hemispherectomy-the Johns Hopkins Experience: 1968 to 1996," *Pediatrics*, 1997 Aug; 100(2 Pt 1): 163-71.

[9] Charles Taylor, *The Ethics of Authenticity* (Cambridge, MA: Harvard University Press, 1992).

[10] Lars Tornstam, "Caring for the Elderly: Introducing the Theory of Gerotranscendence as a Supplementary Frame of Reference for Caring for the Elderly," *Scandinavian Journal of Caring Sciences* 10, no. 3 (1996): 144-150. Lars Tornstam, "Transcendence in Later Life," *Generations: Journal of the American Society on Aging* 23, no. 4 (1999): 10-14.

[11] Erik H Erikson, *Childhood and Society* (New York: WW Norton & Company, 1993). Erik H. Erikson, *Identity and the Life Cycle*. (New York: WW Norton & Company, 1994).

[12] David Gutmann, *Reclaimed Powers: Men and Women in Later Life* (Evanston, IL: Northwestern University Press, 1994).

[13] Irvin Yalom, *Existential Psychotherapy* (New York: Basic Books, 1980).

[14] N. Rogers et al., *Person-Centered & Experiential Psychotherapies* 11, no. 1 (2012): 31-47, p. 43.

[15] A 19th century poet and humanist, Whitman lived from 1819 to 1892.

[16] For example, "Old Age's Lambent Peaks," "Twilight," "Memories," "To Get the Final Lilt of Songs," "Continuities," and "Thanks in Old Age," from, Walt Whitman, *Leaves of Grass* (in the public domain, 1891-1892).

[17] Matthew Ignoffo, "Cosmic Consciousness," J.R. LeMaster and Donald D. Kummings, eds., *Walt Whitman: An Encyclopedia* (New York: Garland Publishing, 1998), pp. 151-152.

[18] Walt Whitman, "Queries to My Seventieth Year," *Leaves of Grass* (in the public domain, 1891-1892).

[19] Carl G. Jung, *Mysterium Coniunctionis: An Inquiry into the Separation and Synthesis of Psychic Opposites in Alchemy* (2nd ed., Vol. 14). Trans. R. F. C. Hull, (Princeton, NJ: Princeton University Press, 1970), p. 42, p. 223.

[1] Dorothy Law Nolte and Rachel Harris. *Children Learn What They Live: Parenting to Inspire Values* (New York, NY: Workman Publishing, 1998): vi-vii.

[2] Helen Keller (born June 27, 1880 – died June 1, 1968), *"The Story of My Life"* (in the public domain, 1904): p. 3.

[3] American Foundation for the Blind, "Helen Keller's Books, Essays, and Speeches," *AFB American Foundation for the Blind*; accessed 22 June 2023, https://www.afb.org/about-afb/history/helen-keller/books-essays-speeches. Britannica, The Editors of Encyclopedia. "Helen Keller," *Encyclopedia Britannica*, 30 Nov. 2022; accessed 24 February 2023 at https://www.britannica.com/biography/Helen-Keller.

[4] See respectively, works by Studs Terkel, ed., *Working: People Talk About What They Do All Day and How They Feel About What They Do* (New York, NY: The New Press, 1974); Bernice L. Neugarten, *The Meanings of Age: Selected Papers* (Chicago, IL: University of Chicago Press); and, Dave Isay, ed., (2007). *Listening Is an Act of Love: A Celebration of American Life from the StoryCorps Project* (New York, NY: Penguin, 2007).

[5] For example, see works by, Joanna Bornat, "Oral History," *Qualitative Research Practice* (2004): 34-47. Bradley J. Fisher, "The Essence of a Life: Life Histories as a Method for Generating Images of Successful Aging," *Teaching Sociology* (1991): 21-27. Mary Ligon, Katie Ehlman, Gabriele Moriello, and E. Ayn Welleford, "Oral History in the Classroom: Fostering Positive Attitudes Toward Older Adults and the Aging Process," *Journal of Aging, Humanities, and the Arts* 3, no. 1 (2009): 59-72. Sandra L. McGuire, Diane A. Klein, and Donna Couper, "Aging Education: A National Imperative," *Educational Gerontology* 31, no. 6 (2005): 443-460.

[6] Karen M. Van Leeuwen, Miriam S. Van Loon, Fenna A. Van Nes, Judith E. Bosmans, Henrica C.W. De Vet, Johannes C.F. Ket, Guy A.M. Widdershoven, and Raymond W.J.G. Ostelo, "What Does Quality of Life Mean to Older Adults? A Thematic Synthesis," *PloS one* 14, no. 3 (2019): e0213263.

[7] M. F. Chan et al., *Health & Social Care in the Community* 21, no. 5 (2013): 545-553. Julia Twigg and Wendy Martin. "The Challenge of Cultural Gerontology," *The Gerontologist* 55, no. 3 (2015): 353-359.

[8] Christopher Booker, *The Seven Basic Plots: Why We Tell Stories* (London: Continuum, 2004).

[9] Thomas Gilovich, Victoria Husted Medvec, and Kenneth Savitsky, "The Spotlight Effect in Social Judgment: An Egocentric Bias in Estimates of the Salience of One's Own Actions and Appearance," *Journal of Personality and Social Psychology* 78, no. 2 (2000): 211-222.

[10] See the reports of Donald E. Gibson and Lisa A. Barron, "Exploring the Impact of Role Models on Older Employees," *Career Development International* 8, no. 4 (2003): pp. 198-209. Penelope Lockwood, Alison L. Chasteen, and Carol Wong, "Age and Regulatory Focus Determine Preferences for Health-Related Role Models," *Psychology and Aging* 20, no. 3 (2005): 376-389. Daniela S. Jopp, Seojung Jung, Amanda K. Damarin, Sheena Mirpuri, and Dario Spini, "Who Is Your Successful Aging Role Model?," *Journals of Gerontology Series B: Psychological Sciences and Social Sciences* 72, no. 2 (2017): 237-247.

[11] Helen Keller, *Optimism: An Essay* (in the public domain, 1903): pp. 13-14.

[12] Anonymous, "Confidently Climb the Stair," May 3, 1950, *Daily Item* (Sunbury, PA); used with permission. Photograph of newspaper clipping from the Helen Keller Digital Archive maintained by the American Foundation for the Blind, "Scrapbook entitled "Scrapbook of Helen Keller and The Blind. Book XXXVII." Created by Rebecca Mack c... May 3, 1950;" Accessed, April 9, 2021, at https://www.afb.org/HelenKellerArchive?a=d&d=A-HK05-B279-BK03-001.1.12&srpos=2&e=-------en-20--1--txt--I+suppose+that+I+age------3-7-6-5-3--------------0-1; Copyright © American Foundation for the Blind, Helen Keller Archive; used with permission.

[13] Peter Armenti, ""For There Is Always Light": Amanda Gorman's Inaugural Poem "The Hill We Climb" Delivers Message of Unity"," June 19, 2023, *Library of Congress Blog*; accessed April 4, 2021, at https://blogs.loc.gov/catbird/2021/01/for-there-is-always-light-amanda-gormans-inaugural-poem-the-hill-we-climb-delivers-message-of-unity/

CHAPTER THREE – THE PAST IS PROLOGUE TO THE FUTURE

[1] William Shakespeare, "Second Part of Henry IV," *The Complete Works of William Shakespeare* (this work is in the public domain, first published in London, 1623): Earl of Warwick to King Henry the Fourth, Act 3, Scene 1.

[2] William Shakespeare, "The Tempest," *The Complete Works of William Shakespeare* (this work is in the public domain, first published in London, 1610-1611): Antonio to Sebastian, Act 2, Scene 1.

[3] Irvin D. Yalom, *Existential Psychotherapy* (New York: Basic Books, 1980). Also see, Dan P. McAdams, "The Psychology of Life Stories," *Review of General Psychology* 5, no. 2 (2001): 100-122. Dan P. McAdams, "The Redemptive Self: Narrative Identity in America Today," in Denise R. Beike, James M. Lampinen, and Douglas A. Behrend (eds.), *The Self and Memory* (New York, NY: Psychology Press, 2004): 95-115.

[4] Faith Gibson, *Reminiscence and Life Story Work: A Practice Guide* (London: Jessica Kingsley Publishers, 2011). Susan Nathan, Laura L. Fiore, Stephanie Saunders, Sandra O. Vilbrun-Bruno PA-C, Kate LM Hinrichs, Marcus D. Ruopp, Andrea Wershof Schwartz, and Jennifer Moye, "My Life, My Story: Teaching Patient Centered Care Competencies for Older Adults Through Life Story Work." *Gerontology & Geriatrics Education* 43, no. 2 (2022): 225-238.

[5] For example, Dan P. McAdams, *The Stories We Live By: Personal Myths and the Making of the Self* (New York, NY: Guilford Press, 1993). Dan P. McAdams, Ruthellen Ed Josselson, and Amia Ed Lieblich, *Identity and Story: Creating Self in Narrative* (Washington, DC: American Psychological Association, 2006). Dan P. McAdams, *Personal Narratives and Life Story* (Cambridge MA: Harvard University Press, 2008).

[6] Dan P. McAdams, "The Psychology of Life Stories," *Review of General Psychology* 5, no. 2 (2001): 100-122. Dan P. McAdams, "Identity and the Life Story," in, Robyn Fivush and Catherine A. Haden, eds., *Autobiographical Memory and the Construction of a Narrative Self* (New York, Psychology Press, 2003): 203-224. Dan P. McAdams and Kate C. McLean, "Narrative Identity," *Current Directions in Psychological Science* 22, no. 3 (2013): 233–238.

[7] For example, see works by Wendy Bottero, "Practising Family History: 'Identity' as a Category of Social Practice," *The British Journal of Sociology* 66, no. 3 (2015): 534-556. Janet Carsten, ed., *Cultures of Relatedness: New Approaches to the Study of Kinship* (New York, NY: Cambridge University Press, 2000). Janet Carsten, *After Kinship*. Vol. 2. (New York, NY: Cambridge University Press, 2004). Karla B. Hackstaff, "Family Genealogy: A Sociological Imagination Reveals Intersectional Relations," *Sociology Compass* 4, no. 8 (2010): 658-672. Donald E. Polkinghorne, "Narrative and Self-Concept," *Journal of Narrative and Life History* 1, no. 2-3 (1991): 135-153. Peter Wade, *Race and Ethnicity in Latin America: How the East India Company Shaped the Modern Multinational (Edition 2)* (London: Pluto Press, 2010). Paul Whitinui, "Indigenous Autoethnography: Exploring, Engaging, and Experiencing "Self" as a Native Method of Inquiry," *Journal of Contemporary Ethnography* 43, no. 4 (2014): 456-487.

[8] Patrick Colm Hogan, *The Mind and Its Stories: Narrative Universals and Human Emotion* (New York, NY: Cambridge University Press, 2003). See also, Patrick Colm Hogan, *Affective Narratology: The Emotional Structure of Stories* (Lincoln, NE: University of Nebraska Press, 2011). Patrick Colm Hogan, *Literature and Moral Feeling: Cognitive Poetics of Ethics, Narrative, and Empathy* (New York, NY: Cambridge University Press, 2022).

[9] Ben Uribe-Cruz, "Stories of Ancestors: Personal Communication with Dean VonDras" (May 24-27, 2021).

[10] Eileen Johnson, "Life story Essay: Personal Communication with Dean VonDras" (May 23, 2021).

[11] Robert N. Butler, "The Life Review: An Interpretation of Reminiscence in the Aged," *Psychiatry* 26, no. 1 (1963): 65-76.

[12] Myrna I. Lewis and Robert N. Butler, "Life-review Therapy. Putting Memories to Work in Individual and Group Psychotherapy." *Geriatrics* 29, no. 11 (1974): 165-173.

[13] Fiona Macleod, Lesley Storey, Teresa Rushe, and Katrina McLaughlin, "Towards an Increased Understanding of Reminiscence Therapy for People with Dementia: A Narrative Analysis," *Dementia* (2020): 1471301220941275.

235

[14] See works by, Hsiu-Fang Hsieh and Jing-Jy Wang, "Effect of Reminiscence Therapy on Depression in Older Adults: A Systematic Review," *International Journal of Nursing Studies* 40, no. 4 (2003): 335-345. Bob Woods, Laura O'Philbin, Emma M. Farrell, Aimee E. Spector, and Martin Orrell, "Reminiscence Therapy for Dementia," *Cochrane Database of Systematic Reviews* 3 (2018). Hsin-Yen Yen and Li-Jung Lin, "A Systematic Review of Reminiscence Therapy for Older Adults in Taiwan," *Journal of Nursing Research* 26, no. 2 (2018): 138-150.

[15] Michael White, Made Wijaya, Michael Kingsley White, and David Epston, *Narrative Means to Therapeutic Ends*, (New York: WW Norton & Company, 1990).

[16] Paula J. Gardner and Jennifer M. Poole, "One Story at a Time: Narrative Therapy, Older adults, and Addictions," *Journal of Applied Gerontology* 28, no. 5 (2009): 600-620.

[17] P. J. Gardner and J. M. Poole: p. 610.

[18] Katrina G. Wellborn and Dean D. VonDras, "A Selective Review and Content Analysis of Narrative and Life story Work with Older Adults," Poster Presented at the *Academic Excellence Symposium*, University of Wisconsin-Green Bay (2021, May).

[19] For example, see reports by, Jennifer N. Auxier, Sian Roberts, Lauren Laing, Lee Finch, Sara Tung, and Lillian Hung, "An Appreciative Inquiry into Older Adults' Pain Experience in Long Term Care Facilities: A Pain Education Initiative," *International Practice Development Journal* 10, no. 1 (2020). M. F. Chan et al., *Health & Social Care in the Community* 21, no. 5 (2013): 545-553. Sanne Jannick Kuipers, Jane Murray Cramm, and Anna Petra Nieboer, "The Importance of Patient-Centered Care and Co-Creation of Care for Satisfaction with Care and Physical and Social Well-Being of Patients with Multi-Morbidity in the Primary Care Setting," *BMC Health Services Research* 19, no. 1 (2019): 1-9. Lewis Mehl-Madrona, Patrick McFarlane, and Barbara Mainguy, "Effects of a Life Story Interview on the Physician–Patient Relationship with Chronic Pain Patients in a Primary Care Setting," *The Journal of Alternative and Complementary Medicine* 27, no. 8 (2021): 688-696.

[20] Karen M. Van Leeuwen et al., *PloS one* 14, no. 3 (2019): e0213263.

[21] For example, see reports by, Jennifer N. Auxier, Sian Roberts, Lauren Laing, Lee Finch, Sara Tung, and Lillian Hung, "An Appreciative Inquiry into Older Adults' Pain Experience in Long Term Care Facilities: A Pain Education Initiative," *International Practice Development Journal* 10, no. 1 (2020). M. F. Chan et al., *Health & Social Care in the Community* 21, no. 5 (2013): 545-553. Sanne Jannick Kuipers, Jane Murray Cramm, and Anna Petra Nieboer, "The Importance of Patient-Centered Care and Co-Creation of Care for Satisfaction with Care and Physical and Social Well-Being of Patients with Multi-Morbidity in the Primary Care Setting," *BMC Health Services Research* 19, no. 1 (2019): 1-9. Moon F. Chan, Sze E. Ng, Adrian Tien, Roger C. Man Ho, and Jeff Thayala, "A Randomised Controlled Study to Explore the Effect of Life Story Review on Depression in Older Chinese in Singapore," *Health & Social Care in the Community* 21, no. 5 (2013): 545-553.

[22] Natalie Joseph-Williams, Glyn Elwyn, and Adrian Edwards, "Knowledge is Not Power for Patients: A Systematic Review and Thematic Synthesis of Patient-Reported Barriers and Facilitators to Shared Decision Making," *Patient Education and Counseling* 94, no. 3 (2014): 291-309. Christina Radl-Karimi, Dorthe Susanne Nielsen, Morten Sodemann, Paul Batalden, and Christian von Plessen, ""When I Feel Safe, I Dare to Open Up": Immigrant and Refugee Patients' Experiences with Coproducing Healthcare," *Patient Education and Counseling* 105, no. 7 (2022): 2338-2345.

[23] Mary Clark Moschella, "Spiritual Autobiography and Older Adults," *Pastoral Psychology* 60, no. 1 (2011): 95-98.

[24] Emily L. Mroz, Susan Bluck, Shubam Sharma, and Hsiao-wen Liao, "Loss in the Life Story: Remembering Death and Illness Across Adulthood," *Psychological Reports* 123, no. 1 (2020): 97-123.

[25] Cecelia L. Thomas and Harriet L. Cohen, "Understanding Spiritual Meaning Making with Older Adults." *Journal of Theory Construction & Testing* 10, no. 2 (2006).

[26] See for example, research by Farida K. Ejaz, Miriam Rose, and Brian Polk, "Evaluating Nursing Home Resident and Staff Experiences With a Life Story Program," *Journal of Applied Gerontology* 41, no. 1 (2022): 124-133. Elise J. Kenter, Winifred A. Gebhardt, Irene Lottman, Mariët van Rossum, Margreet Bekedam, and Mathilde R. Crone, "The Influence of Life Events on Physical Activity Patterns of Dutch Older Adults: A Life History Method," *Psychology & Health* 30, no. 6 (2015): 627-651. L. Mehl-Madrona et al., *Journal of Alternative and Complementary Medicine* 27, no. 8 (2021): 688-696.

[27] Tess Knight, Helen Skouteris, Mardie Townsend, and Merrilyn Hooley, "The Act of Giving: A Pilot and Feasibility Study of the My Life Story Programme Designed to Foster Positive Mental Health and Well-being in Adolescents and Older Adults," *International Journal of Adolescence and Youth* 22, no. 2 (2017): 165-178. Teresa Wills and Mary Rose Day, "Valuing the Person's Story: Use of Life Story Books in a Continuing Care Setting," *Clinical Interventions in Aging* 3, no. 3 (2008): 547-552.

[28] Xue Bai, Daniel W.H. Ho, Karen Fung, Lily Tang, Moon He, Kim Wan Young, Florence Ho, and Timothy Kwok, "Effectiveness of a Life Story Work Program on Older Adults with Intellectual Disabilities," *Clinical Interventions in Aging* 9 (2014): 1865-1872. Anna Gaughan, Bob Woods, Ponnusamy Subramaniam, Steve Milton, Jean Tottie, Gillian Drummond, John Shaw et al., *Life Story Work with People with Dementia: Ordinary Lives, Extraordinary People* (London: Jessica Kingsley Publishers, 2016).

[29] Consuelo Jiminez Underwood, "Life Story Interview with Dean D. VonDras," April 4, 2021.

[30] Consuelo Jimenez Underwood, *Run, Jane, Run!* (Smithsonian American Art Museum, 2004).

[31] Kate Morrissey, "Last Iconic 'Immigrant Crossing Sign' Disappears," February 9, 2018, *The San Diego Union-Tribune*. Accessed May 6, 2021 at https://www.sandiegouniontribune.com/news/immigration/sd-me-immigration-sign-20180208-story.htm

[32] Courtney Lindwall, "Weaving Beauty into the Borderlands," September 16, 2019, *onEarth*. Accessed May 18, 2021 at https://www.nrdc.org/onearth/weaving-beauty-borderlands

CHAPTER FOUR – TRANSITIONS AND EXISTENTIAL CONCERNS THROUGHOUT THE LIFE-COURSE

[1] William James, *The Principles of Psychology* (New York, NY: William Holt and Company, 1890).

[2] See works by Erik H. Erikson, *The Life Cycle Completed. Extended Version* (New York, NY: W.W. Norton & Co., 1997); and, Jean Piaget and Barbel Inhelder, *The Psychology of the Child* (New York, NY: Basic Books, 2008).

[3] Sven Hartman, "Children Searching for a Philosophy of Life," in Jari Ristiniemi, Geir Skeie and Karin Sporre, eds., *Challenging Life: Existential Questions as a Resource for Education* (Münster: Waxmann, 2018): 21-45. Richard D. Logan, "A Reconceptualization of Erikson's Theory: The Repetition of Existential and Instrumental Themes," *Human Development* 29, no. 3 (1986): 125-136. Ingrid Pramling and Eva Johansson, "Existential Questions in Early Childhood Programs in Sweden: Teachers' Conceptions and Children's Experience," In *Child and Youth Care Forum*, vol. 24, no. 2 (Kluwer Academic Publishers Human Sciences Press, 1995): 125-146.

[4] Molly Zhou and David Brown, "Educational Learning Theories," *GALILEO Open Learning Materials*, 2017: Table 8.2.1: "Psychosocial Identity Development Stages, Virtues, and Crisis." Retrieved September 19, 2023 from https://oer.galileo.usg.edu/education-textbooks/1; Also see, Zelda Gillian Knight, "A Proposed Model of Psychodynamic Psychotherapy Linked to Erik Erikson's Eight Stages of Psychosocial Development," *Clinical Psychology & Psychotherapy* 24, no. 5 (2017): 1047-1058. R. D. Logan, *Human Development* 29, no. 3 (1986): 125-136.

[5] Susan Engle, *The Stories Children Tell: Making Sense of the Narratives of Childhood* (New York, NY: Henry Holt and Company, 1995). Evelyn G. Pitcher and Ernst Prelinger, *Children Tell Stories* (Madison, CT: International Universities Press, 1963).

[6] For example, see reports by, Nancy Darling and Laurence Steinberg, "Parenting Style as Context: An Integrative Model," In Brett Laursen and Rita Zakauskiene, eds., *Interpersonal Development* (New York, NY: Routledge, 2017): pp. 161-170; and, Terry Ng-Knight, Katherine H. Shelton, Lucy Riglin, I. C. McManus, Norah Frederickson, and Frances Rice, "A Longitudinal Study of Self-Control at the Transition to Secondary School: Considering the Role of Pubertal Status and Parenting," *Journal of Adolescence* 50 (2016): 44-55.

[7] Okechukwu Stephen Chukwudeh and Akpovire Oduaran, "Liminality and Child Labour: Experiences of School Aged Working Children with Implications for Community Education in Africa," *Social Sciences* 10, no. 3 (2021): 93.

[8] Brett Zyromski, Colette T. Dollarhide, Yahyahan Aras, Sarah Geiger, J. P. Oehrtman, and Halley Clarke. "Beyond Complex Trauma: An Existential View of Adverse Childhood Experiences," *The Journal of Humanistic Counseling* 57, no. 3 (2018): 156-172.

[9] Peter W. Gurney, *Self-esteem in Children with Special Educational Needs* (New York, NY: Routledge, 2018).

[10] For example, see reports by, Christine A. Christle and Mitchell L. Yell, "Preventing Youth Incarceration Through Reading Remediation: Issues and Solutions," *Reading & Writing Quarterly* 24, no. 2 (2008): 148-176; and, Margaret E. Shippen, David E. Houchins, Steven A. Crites, Nicholas C. Derzis, and Dashaunda Patterson, "An Examination of the Basic Reading Skills of Incarcerated Males," *Adult Learning* 21, no. 3-4 (2010): 4-12.

[11] M. Zhou and D. Brown, "Educational Learning Theories," 2015: Table 8.2.1. Also see, R. D. Logan, *Human Development* 29, no. 3 (1986): 125-136.

[12] Timothy Milton Bogen, *Patterns of Developmental Change in Formal Characteristics of Stories Children Tell* (Ann Arbor, MI: University of Michigan, 1982). S. Engle, *The Stories Children Tell: Making Sense of the Narratives of Childhood* (1995). E. G. Pitcher and E. Prelinger, *Children Tell Stories* (1963).

[13] J. Ellsworth, "Addressing Existential Dread," *Gifted* 147 (2008): 26-29; Douglas J. Hacker, "An Existential View of Adolescence," *The Journal of Early Adolescence* 14, no. 3 (1994): 300-327.

[14] M. Zhou and D. Brown, "Educational Learning Theories," 2015: Table 8.2.1. Also see Mary Andrews, "The Existential Crisis," *Behavioral Development Bulletin* 21, no. 1 (2016): 104. R. D. Logan, *Human Development* 29, no. 3 (1986): 125-136. Michael J. Maxwell and Sharon Gayle, "Counseling Adolescent Existential Issues," *Vistas: Ideas and Research You Can Use* 27 (2013): 1-10.

[15] Jefferson A. Singer, "Narrative Identity and Meaning Making Across the Adult Lifespan: An Introduction," *Journal of Personality* 72, no. 3 (2004): 437-460. Jefferson A. Singer and Susan Bluck, "New Perspectives on Autobiographical Memory: The Integration of Narrative Processing and Autobiographical Reasoning," *Review of General Psychology* 5, no. 2 (2001): 91-99.

[16] See reports by Craig M. Hales, Margaret D. Carroll, Cheryl D. Fryar, and Cynthia L. Ogden, "Prevalence of Obesity Among Adults and Youth: United States, 2015–2016," (2017); National Center for Health Statistics (U.S.), "Health, United States, 2019." (2021); and, Megan E. Patrick, Yvonne M. Terry-McElrath, Stephanie T. Lanza, Justin Jager, John E. Schulenberg, and Patrick M. O'Malley, "Shifting Age of Peak Binge Drinking Prevalence: Historical Changes in Normative Trajectories Among Young Adults Aged 18 to 30," *Alcoholism: Clinical and Experimental Research* 43, no. 2 (2019): 287-298.

[17] William G. Perry Jr., *Forms of Intellectual and Ethical Development in the College Years: A Scheme. Jossey-Bass Higher and Adult Education Series*. San Francisco, CAL Jossey-Bass Publishers, 1999).

[18] See works respectively by, M. Zhou and D. Brown, "Educational Learning Theories," 2015: Table 8.2.1. Also see, R. D. Logan, *Human Development* 29, no. 3 (1986): 125-136; and, Kristin L. Sommer, Roy F. Baumeister, and Tyler F. Stillman "The Construction of Meaning from Life Events: Empirical Studies of Personal Narratives," in P. T. Wong, ed., *The Human Quest for Meaning* (New York, NY: Routledge, 2013): 297-313.

[19] Dan P. McAdams and Kate C. McLean, "Narrative identity," *Current Directions in Psychological Science* 22, no. 3 (2013): 233-238. Theodore E.A. Waters and Robyn Fivush, "Relations Between Narrative Coherence, Identity, and Psychological Well-being in Emerging Adulthood," *Journal of Personality* 83, no. 4 (2015): 441-451.

[20] Carl G. Jung, "The Stages of Life," *Volume 8 of the Collected Works of C. G. Jung*, 2nd ed., (Princeton, NJ: Princeton University Press, 1969); Bernice L. Neugarten, "Adult Personality: A Developmental View," *Human Development* 9, no. 1/2 (1966): 61-73.

[21] M. Zhou and D. Brown, "Educational Learning Theories," 2015: Table 8.2.1. Also see, R. D. Logan, *Human Development* 29, no. 3 (1986): 125-136. John W. Osborne, "Commentary on Retirement, Identity, and Erikson's Developmental Stage Model," *Canadian Journal on Aging/La Revue Canadienne du Vieillissement* 28, no. 4 (2009): 295-301.

22 Federico Gomez-Bernal, Elizabeth N. Madva, Judith Puckett, Hermioni L. Amonoo, Rachel A. Millstein, and Jeff C. Huffman, "Relationships Between Life Stressors, Health Behaviors, and Chronic Medical Conditions in Mid-life Adults: A Narrative Review," *Psychosomatics* 60, no. 2 (2019): 153-163. Dan P. McAdams, "The Life Narrative at Midlife," *New Directions for Child and Adolescent Development* 145 (2014): 57-69. Dan P. McAdams and Jen Guo, "Narrating the Generative Life," *Psychological Science* 26, no. 4 (2015): 475-483. Hollen N. Reischer, Laura J. Roth, Jorge A. Villarreal, and Dan P. McAdams, "Self-transcendence and Life stories of Humanistic Growth Among Late-Midlife Adults," *Journal of Personality* 89, no. 2 (2021): 305-324.

23 Lars Tornstam, "Maturing into Gerotranscendence" *Journal of Transpersonal Psychology* 43, no. 2 (2011); Lars Tornstam, *Gerotranscendence, A Developmental Theory of Positive Aging,* (New York, NY: Springer Publishing Company, Inc., 2005). Also see the stage extension proposed in by Erik H. Erikson and Joan M. Erikson, "The Life Cycle Completed: Extended Version," (New York, NY: W.W. Norton, 1998).

24 Jack J. Bauer and Sun W. Park, "Growth is Not Just for the Young: Growth Narratives, Eudaimonic Resilience, and the Aging Self," in P. S. Fry and C. L. M. Keyes, eds. *New Frontiers in Resilient Aging: Life-strengths and Well-being in Late Life* (Cambridge University Press, 2010): 60-89. D. P. McAdams and B. D. Olson, B.D., "Personality Development: Continuity and Change Over the Life Course," *Annual Review of Psychology 61* (2010): 517-542. Cora Rice and Monisha Pasupathi, "Reflecting on Self-relevant Experiences: Adult Age Differences," *Developmental Psychology* 46, no. 2 (2010): 479-490.

25 Chris Lo, "A Developmental Perspective on Existential Distress and Adaptation to Advanced Disease," *Psycho-Oncology* 27, no. 11 (2018): 2657-2660. Brianne van Rhyn, Alex Barwick, and Michelle Donelly, "Embodied Experiences and Existential Reflections of the Oldest Old," *Journal of Aging Studies* 61 (2022): 101028.

26 Brent C. Miller and Diana Gerard, "Family Influences on the Development of Creativity in Children: An Integrative Review," *Family Coordinator* (1979): 295-312.

27 For example, see works by Bjarne S. Funch, "Art, Emotion, and Existential Well-Being," *Journal of Theoretical and Philosophical Psychology* 41, no. 1 (2021): 5; Tim Newsome-Ward and Jenna Ng, "Between Subjectivity and Flourishing: Creativity and Game Design as Existential Meaning," *Games and Culture* (2021): 15554120211048015; and, Rotem Perach and Arnaud Wisman, "Can Creativity Beat Death? A Review and Evidence on the Existential Anxiety Buffering Functions of Creative Achievement," *The Journal of Creative Behavior* 53, no. 2 (2019): 193-210.

28 Dean D. VonDras, "Victoria Poullette Jicha Personal Communication with Dean D. VonDras" (November 6, 2020).

29 Victoria Poullette Jicha, "If I Only Knew Then What I Know Now," *Flute Talk* (December, 2021).

[30] E. H. Erikson and J. M. Erikson, "The Life Cycle Completed: Extended Version," (1998).

[31] Herman Hesse, *Demian* (1918, in the public domain).

CHAPTER FIVE – SUPPORTING CAST AND SURROUNDING CHARACTERS: KITH AND KIN

[1] Lawrence J. Epstein, *George Burns: An American Life* (Jefferson, NC: McFarland & Company, 2011).

[2] For further reading see works by Arthur Asa Berger, "Humor: An Introduction," *American Behavioral Scientist* 30, no. 3 (1987): 6-15; Ted Cohen, *Jokes: Philosophical Thoughts on Joking Matters* (Chicago, IL: University of Chicago Press, 1999); Victor Raskin (ed.), *The Primer of Humor Research*, Vol. 8 (New York, NY: Walter de Gruyter, 2008).

[3] Mary Douglas, "Do Dogs Laugh? A Cross-Cultural Approach to Body Symbolism," *Journal of Psychosomatic Research* 15, no. 4 (1971): 387-390.

[4] Geert Hofstede, Gert Jan Hofstede, and Michael Minkov, *Cultures and Organizations: Software of the Mind, Third Edition* (New York, NY: McGraw-Hill, 2010).

[5] Richard A. Shweder, *Thinking Through Cultures: Expeditions in Cultural Psychology* (Cambridge, MA: Harvard University Press, 1991); Richard Shweder, Manamohan Mahapatra, and Jerome G. Miller, "Culture and Development," in J. Kagan and S. Lamb, eds., *The Emergence of Morality in Young Children* (Chicago, IL: University Chicago Press,1987): 1-83.

[6] Jon Haidt, "The Emotional Dog and Its Rational Tail: A Social Intuitionist Approach to Moral Judgment," *Psychological Review, 108(4)*, 2001: 814-834.

[7] See works by, Gerald Jones, *"Honey I'm Home!: Sitcoms: Selling the American Dream,"* (New York, NY: Macmillan, 1993); Anthony J. Marsella, "Some Reflections on Potential Abuses of Psychology's Knowledge and Practices," *Psychological Studies* 54, no. 1 (2009): 23-27.

[8] Andre Cavalcante, "Anxious Displacements: The Representation of Gay Parenting on Modern Family and The New Normal and the Management of Cultural Anxiety," *Television & New Media* 16, no. 5 (2015): 454-471. Jillian Fabiano, "7 Times *Black-ish* Taught Us About Social Movements," February 15, 2022, *E-News*, E-Online. Accessed, March 1, 2023 at https://www.eonline.com/news/1318939/7-times-black-ish-taught-us-about-social-movements. Joanne R. Gilbert "Performing Marginality: Comedy, Identity, and Cultural Critique," *Text and Performance Quarterly* 17, no. 4 (1997): 317-330. Sylvia Henneberg, "Rewriting the How-To of Parenting: What Is Really Modern about ABC's Modern Family," *Journal of Interdisciplinary Feminist Thought* 9, no. 1 (2016): 1. Jacques Rothman, "'Send in the (Gay) Clowns': Will & Grace and Modern Family as 'Sensibly Queer'," *Acta Academica* 45, no. 4 (2013): 40-83. Gina H. Salinas, "From Good Times to Blackish: A Content Analysis of the Portrayal of African American Women Through the American Television Sitcom" (PhD diss., California State University, Sacramento, 2021).

[9] For example, IMDb, "Legends of a Monkey God" (Hanuman Productions, 2018); retrieved April 2, 2022 at https://www.imdb.com/title/tt9298240/; and, IMDb, "Bu Ken Qu Guan Yin aka Avalokiteshvara" (Beijing Spencer Culture & Media, 2013); retrieved April 2, 2022 https://www.imdb.com/title/tt3428458/.

[10] See works by, Anne Birrell, *Chinese Myths* (Austin, TX: University of Texas Press, 2000); John H. Chamberlayne, "The Development of Kuan Yin: Chinese Goddess of Mercy," *Numen* 9, no. Fasc. 1 (1962): 45-52; Edward Theodore Chalmers Werner, *Myths and Legends of China* (North Chelmsford, MA: Courier Corporation, 1994).

[11] See for example, Karen Austin, "Deadly Funny: The Aboriginal Stand-up Comedians Cracking Up Australia," *The Conversation*, March 28, 2017; accessed April 2, 2022 at https://www.abc.net.au/news/2017-03-29/deadly-funny-the-aboriginal-comedians-cracking-up-australia/8396586; Kristina Rose Fagan, *Laughing to Survive, Humour in Contemporary Canadian Native Literature* (PhD diss., University of Toronto, 2001); Kenneth Lincoln, *Indi'n humor: Bicultural Play in Native America* (New York, NY: Oxford University Press, 1993).

[12] Elizabeth C. Vozzola, *Moral Development: Theory and Applications* (New York, NY: Routledge, 2014).

[13] For example, see, A.J. Samuels, "10 African Movies You Need to Watch," *The Culture Trip*, May 12, 2017; access April 2, 2022 at https://theculturetrip.com/africa/articles/10-african-movies-you-need-to-watch/.

[14] For example, Nankap Lamle Elias, and Iliya Ayuba Dauda, "Tarok, Wolof, Mandika Joking Relationships, Humour and Peace Building in Africa," *Journal of Good Governance and Sustainable Development in Africa* 5, no. 1 (2019): 86-95. Katz, Richard Katz, *Boiling Energy: Community Healing Among the Kalahari Kung* (Boston, MA: Harvard University Press, 1982).

[15] Ebenezer Obadare, "State of Travesty: Jokes and the Logic of Socio-Cultural Improvisation in Africa," *Critical African Studies* 2, no. 4 (2010): 92-112.

[16] Liz Medendorp, "The Goldbergs Are a Strangely Familiar Family," October 6, 2015, *PopMatters*, PopMatters Media. Accessed March 2, 2023 at https://www.popmatters.com/the-goldbergs-the-complete-second-season-2495483155.html

[17] For example, see, Karen L. Fingerman, Karl A. Pillemer, Merril Silverstein, and J. Jill Suitor, "The Baby Boomers' Intergenerational Relationships," *The Gerontologist* 52, no. 2 (2012): 199-209; Ann Goetting, "The Developmental Tasks of Siblingship Over the Life Cycle," *Journal of Marriage and the Family* (1986): 703-714; Maria Schmeeckle and Susan Sprecher, "Widening Circles: Interactive Connections Between Immediate Family and Larger Social Networks," in, Anita L. Vangelisti, ed., *The Routledge Handbook of Family Communication* (New York, NY: Routledge, 2012): 314-330.

[18] Richard Schulz, Alison T. O'Brien, Jamila Bookwala, and Kathy Fleissner, "Psychiatric and Physical Morbidity Effects of Dementia Caregiving: Prevalence, Correlates, and Causes," *The Gerontologist* 35, no. 6 (1995): 771-791; Richard Schulz, Paul Visintainer, and Gail M. Williamson, "Psychiatric and Physical Morbidity Effects of Caregiving," *Journal of Gerontology* 45, no. 5 (1990): P181-P191.

[19] See for example reports by, Betty J. Kramer, "Gain in the Caregiving Experience: Where Are We? What Next?," *The Gerontologist* 37, no. 2 (1997): 218-232; Richard Schulz and Paula R. Sherwood, "Physical and Mental Health Effects of Family Caregiving," *Journal of Social Work Education* 44, no. sup3 (2008): 105-113; Shanshan Wang, Daphne Sze Ki Cheung, Angela Yee Man Leung, and Patricia M. Davidson, "Factors Associated with Caregiving Appraisal of Informal Caregivers: A Systematic Review," *Journal of Clinical Nursing* 29, no. 17-18 (2020): 3201-3221.

[20] Andrew Cherlin and Frank F. Furstenberg, Jr., "Styles and Strategies of Grandparenting," In V. L. Bengtson and J. F. Robertson, eds., *Grandparenthood* (Newbury Park, CA: Sage Publications, Inc., 1985): pp. 97-116; Merril Silverstein and Anne Marenco, "How Americans Enact the Grandparent Role Across the Family Life Course," *Journal of Family Issues* 22, no. 4 (2001): 493-522.

21 For example, see works by, Carlo Cristini and Marcello Cesa-Bianchi, "Culture, Creativity and Quality of Life in Old Age," *Italian Studies on Quality of Life* (2019): 243-253; Einat Shuper Engelhard, "Free-Form Dance as an Alternative Interaction for Adult Grandchildren and Their Grandparents," *Frontiers in Psychology* 11 (2020): 542; Kathleen Mundell, "Elderhood Arts," in J. Kay, ed., *The Expressive Lives of Elders: Folklore, Art, and Aging* (Bloomington, IN: Indiana University Press, 2018): 175; Anita Curtis Reyes, Terrence Neville Hays, and Mary M. Read, "Grandparent Tales: Exploring the Intergenerational Transmission of Life Stories Through Photographic Expressive Arts," in T. N. Hays and R. Hussain, eds., *Bridging the Gap between Ideas and Doing Research: Proceedings of the Inaugural Postgraduate Research Conference* (Victoria, AU: Australian College of Educators, 2007): 327-327.

22 For example, see, Maaike Jappens and Jan Van Bavel, "Parental Divorce, Residence Arrangements, and Contact Between Grandchildren and Grandparents," *Journal of Marriage and Family* 78, no. 2 (2016): 451-467.

23 Pedro Javier Castañeda-García, Vanesa Cruz-Santana, Fayna Hernández-Garrido, Paula Díaz-Rodríguez, and Sara Romero-González, "Which Activities Do Great-Grandparents and Great-Grandchildren Share in Family Contexts? An Analysis of a New Intergenerational Relationship," *Anales de Psicología/Annals of Psychology* 37, no. 2 (2021): 265-275.

24 Michael W. Pratt, Joan E. Norris, Shannon Hebblethwaite, and Mary Louise Arnold, "Intergenerational Transmission of Values: Family Generativity and Adolescents' Narratives of Parent and Grandparent Value Teaching," *Journal of Personality* 76, no. 2 (2008): 171-198.

25 Erich Fromm, *The Art of Loving: The Centennial Edition* (New York, NY: A&C Black, 2000).

26 Eva Kahana, Tirth R. Bhatta, Boaz Kahana, and Nirmala Lekhak. "Loving Others: The Impact of Compassionate Love on Later Life Psychological Well-being," *The Journals of Gerontology: Series B* 76, no. 2 (2021): 391-402.

27 Margaret Neiswender Reedy, James E. Birren, and Warner Schaie, "Age and Sex Differences in Satisfying Love Relationships Across the Adult Life Span," *Human Development* 24, no. 1 (1981): 52-66.

28 Robert J. Sternberg, *Love is a Story: A New Theory of Relationships* (Oxford: Oxford University Press, 1999).

29 Robert J. Sternberg, "Love Stories," *Personal Relationships* 3, no. 1 (1996): 59-79.

30 Kaarina Määttä, "How to Learn to Love--How to Guide the Young to Love?," *Education Sciences & Psychology* 17, no. 2 (2010).

31 Scott Wallestad and Dean D. VonDras, "Humanistic Gerontology: Growing Further," Paper Presented at the UWGB Academic Excellence Symposium, May 11, 2020.

32 Sthephany Escandell and Dean D. VonDras, "In the Light and Dark Moments of Aging," Paper Presented at the UWGB Academic Excellence Symposium, April 27, 2020.

[33] Erik H. Erikson, *The Life Cycle Completed. Extended Version* (New York, NY: W.W. Norton & Co., 1997); Irvin Yalom, *Existential Psychotherapy* (New York: Basic Books, 1980).

[34] Joseph M. Champlin, *From Time to Eternity and Back: A Priest's Successful Struggle with Cancer* (Staten Island, NY: Alba House, 2004).

[35] See reviews by Sandra B. Barker and Aaron R. Wolen, "The Benefits of Human–Companion Animal Interaction: A Review," *Journal of Veterinary Medical Education* 35, no. 4 (2008): 487-495; Sarah J. Brodie and Francis C. Biley, "An Exploration of the Potential Benefits of Pet-Facilitated Therapy," *Journal of Clinical Nursing* 8, no. 4 (1999): 329-337; Nancy Gee and Megan K. Mueller, "A Systematic Review of Research on Pet Ownership and Animal Interactions Among Older Adults," *Anthrozoös* 32, no. 2 (2019): 183-207; Shirley D. Hooker, Linda Holbrook Freeman, and Pamela Stewart, "Pet Therapy Research: A Historical Review," *Holistic Nursing Practice* 17, no. 1 (2002): 17-23.

[36] For example, see works by the following: Chelsea G. Himsworth and Melanie Rock, "Pet Ownership, Other Domestic Relationships, and Satisfaction with Life among Seniors: Results from a Canadian National Survey," *Anthrozoös* 26, no. 2 (2013): 295-305; Barker and Wolen (2008); Gee and Mueller (2019); and by, Susan Krieger, *Come, Let Me Guide You: A Life Shared with a Guide Dog* (West Lafayette, IN: Purdue University Press, 2015).

[37] For example, see, Kent LaVoie (LOBO), *Me and You and a Dog Named Boo* (Los Angeles, CA: Sony/ATV Music Publishing, 1971); George Bruns, "A Cowboy Needs a Horse," (Los Angeles, CA: Walt Disney Productions, 1956); JoAnn Jordan, "Animal Songs for Young and Old," *MusicSparks,* October 6, 2011. https://www.music2spark.com/2011/10/03/animal-songs/ The Doubleclicks, *Boundaries (Marzipan the Cat),* (Los Angeles, CA: The Doubleclicks, 2019). https://www.thedoubleclicks.com/music/

[38] Robert Dunsky, Theresa Dunsky, and Mary Elizabeth VonDras, "Personal Communications about the Life and Times of Dr. Milton H. Dunsky, 1932-2020, to Dean D. VonDras" (November, 2020).

[39] See respectively the works, Kenny Clarke and Dizzy Gillespie, *Salt Peanuts* (New York, NY: Guild Records, 1945); and, Leonard Bernstein, Jerome Robbins, Arthur Laurents, Stephen Sondheim, Irwin Kostal, Sid Ramin, Betsi Morrison, et al., *West Side Story: The Original Score* (Hong Kong: Naxos, 2002). https://www.naxosmusiclibrary.com.

[40] Stan Getz and Charlie Byrd, *Jazz Samba* (Los Angeles, CA: MGM/Verve Records, 1962).

[41] Dunsky et al., (November, 2020). This music-animal-human relationship is also alluded to in the existential notions shared by Franz Kafka, in his short story, "Investigations of a Dog" (in, *Franz Kafka: The Complete Stories*, trans. Edwin and Willa Muir (New York: Schocken Books, 1971), pp. 278-316). Writing from the perspective of the dog, and suggestive of the common bond we share with animals, Kafka considers the nature and limits of our understanding, and alludes to how all inquiries and concerns of knowledge are represented within the canine. Similar to our human understanding, in his dog-narrative Kafka notes the mesmerizing power of music and its grandeur. Thus, distinguishing music as an area of higher inquiry, whose knowledge is more observational, systematized, and comprehensive than the dog's scientific explorations of nurture or the satisfaction of one's hunger for food.

[42] Art Linkletter, *Kids Say The Darndest Things!, Illus. by Charles Schulz* (New York, NY: Simon, 1957); Ryan Schwartz, *"Kids Say the Darndest Things, With Tiffany Haddish, Revived at CBS,"* December 17, 2020, *TVLine;* accessed April 15, 2022, at https://tvline.com/2020/12/17/kids-say-the-darndest-things-revival-tiffany-haddish-returning-season-2-cbs/#!

[43] Norman Cousins, *Anatomy of an Illness* (New York, NY: W. W. Norton, 1979).

CHAPTER SIX – ENTER THE MONSTER

[1] Marcus Tullius Cicero, *Letters of Marcus Tullius Cicero, with His Treatises on Friendship and Old Age*, trans. by E. S. Shuckburgh (This work is in the public domain, 1909).

[2] See respectively works by the following: Leonard Hayflick, "Aging: The Reality: "Anti-Aging" Is an Oxymoron," *The Journals of Gerontology Series A: Biological Sciences and Medical Sciences* 59, no. 6 (2004): B573. De Magalhães, João Pedro, Michael Stevens, and Daniel Thornton, "The Business of Anti-Aging Science," *Trends in Biotechnology* 35, no. 11 (2017): 1062-1073. Ji-Kai Liu, "Antiaging Agents: Safe Interventions to Slow Aging and Healthy Life Span Extension," *Natural Products and Bioprospecting* 12, no. 1 (2022): 18. Devin Wahl, Rozalyn M. Anderson, and David G. Le Couteur, "Antiaging Therapies, Cognitive Impairment, and Dementia," *The Journals of Gerontology: Series A* 75, no. 9 (2020): 1643-1652. Arlene Weintraub, *Selling the Fountain of Youth: How the Anti-Aging Industry Made a Disease Out of Getting Old-and Made Billions* (New York: Basic Books, 2010).

[3] Penelope Foretich, "The 5 Stages of Aging: What Seniors and Family Need to Understand," *Online Senior Center*, February 13, 2022. Accessed February 1, 2023 at https://onlineseniorcenter.com/resources/the-5-stages-of-aging/

[4] Allen L. Pelletier, Ledy Rojas-Roldan, and Janis Coffin, "Vision Loss in Older Adults," *American Family Physician* 94, no. 3 (2016): 219-226. Cynthia Owsley, "Aging and Vision," *Vision Research* 51, no. 13 (2011): 1610-1622. Bonnielin K. Swenor, Moon J. Lee, Varshini Varadaraj, Heather E. Whitson, and Pradeep Y. Ramulu, "Aging with Vision Loss: A Framework for Assessing the Impact of Visual Impairment on Older Adults." *The Gerontologist* 60, no. 6 (2020): 989-995.

[5] A. L. Pelletier et al., *American Family Physician* 94, no. 3 (2016).

[6] John E. Crews, Chiu-Fang Chou, Swathi Sekar, and Jinan B. Saaddine, "The Prevalence of Chronic Conditions and Poor Health Among People With and Without Vision Impairment, Aged≥ 65 years, 2010–2014," *American Journal of Ophthalmology* 182 (2017): 18-30. B. K. Swenor et al., *The Gerontologist* 60, no. 6 (2020).

[7] Marlene Chu, "Low Vision Aids, Adaptations, Resources," *Tech-enhanced Life*, September, 14, 2017. Accessed February 2, 2023 at https://www.techenhancedlife.com/articles/low-vision-aids-adaptations-resources. Marlene Chu, "Low Vision App Overview," *Tech-enhanced Life*, September, 10, 2021. Accessed February 2, 2023 at https://www.techenhancedlife.com/citizen-research/low-vision-app-overview.

[8] Michael R. Bowl and Sally J. Dawson, "Age-Related Hearing Loss," *Cold Spring Harbor Perspectives in Medicine* 9, no. 8 (2019): a033217. Lee, Kyu-Yup Lee, "Pathophysiology of Age-Related Hearing Loss (Peripheral and Central)," *Korean Journal of Audiology* 17, no. 2 (2013): 45-49.

[9] Andrea Ciorba, Chiara Bianchini, Stefano Pelucchi, and Antonio Pastore, "The Impact of Hearing Loss on the Quality of Life of Elderly Adults," *Clinical Interventions in Aging* (2012): 159-163. Cynthia D. Mulrow, Christine Aguilar, James E. Endicott, Ramon Velez, Michael R. Tuley, Walter S. Charlip, and Judith A. Hill, "Association Between Hearing Impairment and the Quality of Life of Elderly Individuals," *Journal of the American Geriatrics Society* 38, no. 1 (1990): 45-50.

[10] Richard L. Doty, Paul Shaman, Steven L. Applebaum, Ronita Giberson, Lenore Siksorski, and Lysa Rosenberg, "Smell Identification Ability: Changes with Age," *Science* 226, no. 4681 (1984): 1441-1443. Richard L. Doty and James B. Snow. "Age-related Alterations in Olfactory Structure and Function" in F. Margolis and T. Getchell, eds., *Molecular Neurobiology of the Olfactory System: Molecular, Membranous, and Cytological Studies* (1988): 355-374.

[11] Valentina Parma, Kathrin Ohla, Maria G. Veldhuizen, Masha Y. Niv, Christine E. Kelly, Alyssa J. Bakke, Keiland W. Cooper et al., "More than Smell—COVID-19 is Associated With Severe Impairment of Smell, Taste, and Chemesthesis," *Chemical senses* 45, no. 7 (2020): 609-622. Susan S. Schiffman, "Taste and Smell Losses in Normal Aging and Disease," *JAMA* 278, no. 16 (1997): 1357-1362.

[12] Frank Schieber, "Aging and the Senses," *Handbook of Mental Health and Aging* (New York, NY: Academic Press, 1992): 251-306.

[13] Stefan Lautenbacher, Jan H. Peters, Michael Heesen, Jennifer Scheel, and Miriam Kunz, "Age Changes in Pain Perception: A Systematic-Review and Meta-Analysis of Age Effects on Pain and Tolerance Thresholds," *Neuroscience & Biobehavioral Reviews* 75 (2017): 104-113.

[14] Regina M. Leadley, Nigel Armstrong, Kim J. Reid, Alex Allen, Kate V. Misso, and Jos Kleijnen, "Healthy Aging in Relation to Chronic Pain and Quality of Life in Europe," *Pain Practice* 14, no. 6 (2014): 547-558. Christine Miaskowski, Fiona Blyth, Francesca Nicosia, Mary Haan, Frances Keefe, Alexander Smith, and Christine Ritchie "A Biopsychosocial Model of Chronic Pain for Older Adults," *Pain Medicine* 21, no. 9 (2020): 1793-1805. M. Carrington Reid, Christopher Eccleston, and Karl Pillemer, "Management of Chronic Pain in Older Adults," *BMJ* 350 (2015).

[15] Muyinat Y. Osoba, Ashwini K. Rao, Sunil K. Agrawal, and Anil K. Lalwani, "Balance and Gait in the Elderly: A Contemporary Review," *Laryngoscope Investigative Otolaryngology* 4, no. 1 (2019): 143-153. Scott W. Shaffer and Anne L. Harrison. "Aging of the Somatosensory System: A Translational Perspective," *Physical Therapy* 87, no. 2 (2007): 193-207.

[16] Y. Lajoie and S. P. Gallagher, "Predicting Falls Within the Elderly Community: Comparison of Postural Sway, Reaction Time, the Berg Balance Scale and the Activities-Specific Balance Confidence (ABC) Scale for Comparing Fallers and Non-fallers," *Archives of Gerontology and Geriatrics* 38, no. 1 (2004): 11-26.

[17] Caroline Landelle, Marie Chancel, Caroline Blanchard, Michel Guerraz, and Anne Kavounoudias, "Contribution of Muscle Proprioception to Limb Movement Perception and Proprioceptive Decline with Ageing," *Current Opinion in Physiology* 20 (2021): 180-185.

[18] John Mendoza and Anne Foundas, *Clinical Neuroanatomy: A Neurobehavioral Approach* (New York, NY: Springer Science & Business Media, 2007).

[19] Laurence Z. Rubenstein, "Falls in Older People: Epidemiology, Risk Factors and Strategies for Prevention," *Age and Ageing* 35, no. suppl_2 (2006): ii37-ii41.

[20] Leonard Hayflick, "Theories of Biological Aging," *Experimental Gerontology* 20, no. 3-4 (1985): 145-159. Julia Holmes, *"Aging Differently: Physical Limitations Among Adults Aged 50 Years and Over: United States, 2001-2007. No. 20.* US Department of Health and Human Services, Centers for Disease Control and Prevention, National Center for Health Statistics (2009). Nathan Wetherill Shock, *Normal Human Aging: The Baltimore Longitudinal Study of Aging,* No. 84, US Department of Health and Human Services, Public Health Service, National Institutes of Health, National Institute on Aging, Gerontology Research Center (1984). Anthony A. Vandervoort, "Aging of the Human Neuromuscular System," *Muscle & Nerve: Official Journal of the American Association of Electrodiagnostic Medicine* 25, no. 1 (2002): 17-25.

[21] Walter M. Bortz, "A Conceptual Framework of Frailty: A Review," *The Journals of Gerontology Series A: Biological Sciences and Medical Sciences* 57, no. 5 (2002): M283-M288. Frank Lally and Peter Crome, "Understanding Frailty," *Postgraduate Medical Journal* 83, no. 975 (2007): 16-20.

22 Sidney Katz, "Assessing Self-maintenance: Activities of Daily Living, Mobility, and Instrumental Activities of Daily Living," *Journal of the American Geriatrics Society* 31, no. 12 (1983): 721-727.

23 William J. Strawbridge, Sarah J. Shema, Jennifer L. Balfour, Helen R. Higby, and George A. Kaplan "Antecedents of Frailty Over Three Decades in an Older Cohort," *The Journals of Gerontology Series B: Psychological Sciences and Social Sciences* 53, no. 1 (1998): S9-S16.

24 Centers for Disease Control and Prevention, National Center for Health Statistics. National Vital Statistics System, *Mortality 1999-2020 on CDC WONDER Online Database, Released in 2021.* "Data are from the Multiple Cause of Death Files, 1999-2020, as compiled from data provided by the 57 vital statistics jurisdictions through the Vital Statistics Cooperative Program." Accessed February 2, 2023, at http://wonder.cdc.gov/ucd-icd10.html on February 2, 2023.

25 Healthy Aging Team, "The Top 10 Most Common Chronic Conditions in Older Adults," *National Council on Aging*, April 23, 2021. Accessed on February 2, 2023, at https://www.ncoa.org/age-well-planner/resource/the-top-10-most-common-chronic-conditions-in-older-adults

26 Raquel Lara, Mª Luisa Vázquez, Adelaida Ogallar, and Débora Godoy-Izquierdo, "Optimism and Social Support Moderate the Indirect Relationship Between Self-Efficacy and Happiness Through Mental Health in the Elderly," *Health Psychology Open* 7, no. 2 (2020): 2055102920947905. Jennifer Morozink Boylan, Justin L. Tompkins, and Patrick M. Krueger, "Psychological Well-Being, Education, and Mortality," *Health Psychology* 41, no. 3 (2022): 225-234.

27 Teresa Niccoli and Linda Partridge, "Ageing as a Risk Factor for Disease," *Current Biology* 22, no. 17 (2012): R741-R752.

28 Olvera Alvarez, Hector A., Allison A. Appleton, Christina H. Fuller, Annie Belcourt, and Laura D. Kubzansky, "An Integrated Socio-Environmental Model of Health and Well-being: A Conceptual Framework Exploring the Joint Contribution of Environmental and Social Exposures to Health and Disease Over the Life Span," *Current Environmental Health Reports* 5 (2018): 233-243. Ross C. Brownson, Debra Haire-Joshu, and Douglas A. Luke, "Shaping the Context of Health: A Review of Environmental and Policy Approaches in the Prevention of Chronic Diseases," *Annual Review of Public Health* 27 (2006): 341-370. Linda J. Jones, *The Social Context of Health and Health Work* (London: Bloomsbury Publishing, 1994). Jeanne Miranda, Thomas G. McGuire, David R. Williams, and Philip Wang, "Mental Health in the Context of Health Disparities," *American Journal of Psychiatry* 165, no. 9 (2008): 1102-1108.

29 Editors, "Top 10 Causes of Death," *Fact Sheet, World Health Organization*, December 9, 2020. Accessed February 7, 2023 at https://www.who.int/news-room/fact-sheets/detail/the-top-10-causes-of-death.

[30] Amir A. Sadighi Akha, "Aging and the Immune System: An Overview," *Journal of Immunological Methods* 463 (2018): 21-26. Jennifer E. Graham, Lisa M. Christian, and Janice K. Kiecolt-Glaser. "Stress, Age, and Immune Function: Toward a Lifespan Approach," *Journal of Behavioral Medicine* 29 (2006): 389-400. Donna Ray and Raymond Yung, "Immune Senescence, Epigenetics and Autoimmunity," *Clinical Immunology* 196 (2018): 59-63.

[31] F.C Bennett and A. V. Molofsky, "The Immune System and Psychiatric Disease: A Basic Science Perspective," *Clinical & Experimental Immunology* 197, no. 3 (2019): 294-307. Barbara Dorian and Paul E. Garfinkel, "Stress, Immunity and Illness—A Review," *Psychological Medicine* 17, no. 2 (1987): 393-407.

[32] Peter P. Vitaliano, Richard Schulz, Janice Kiecolt-Glaser, and Igor Grant, "Research on Physiological and Physical Concomitants of Caregiving: Where Do We Go from Here?," *Annals of Behavioral Medicine* 19, no. 2 (1997): 117-123.

[33] Robert S. Baron, Carolyn E. Cutrona, Daniel Hicklin, Daniel W. Russell, and David M. Lubaroff, "Social Support and Immune Function Among Spouses of Cancer Patients," *Journal of Personality and Social Psychology* 59, no. 2 (1990): 344. George S. Everly, Jr., Jeffrey M. Lating, George S. Everly, and Jeffrey M. Lating, "Stress-related Disease: A Review," *A Clinical Guide to the Treatment of the Human Stress Response* (2019): 85-127. Janice K. Kiecolt-Glaser, Phillip T. Marucha, Ana M. Mercado, William B. Malarkey, and Ronald Glaser, "Slowing of Wound Healing by Psychological Stress," *The Lancet* 346, no. 8984 (1995): 1194-1196. Jeanette I. Webster Marketon and Ronald Glaser, "Stress Hormones and Immune Function," *Cellular Immunology* 252, no. 1-2 (2008): 16-26. Jennifer R. Piazza, David M. Almeida, Natalia O. Dmitrieva, and Laura C. Klein, "Frontiers in the Use of Biomarkers of Health in Research on Stress and Aging," *Journals of Gerontology Series B: Psychological Sciences and Social Sciences* 65, no. 5 (2010): 513-525.

[34] Janice K. Kiecolt-Glaser, Lynanne McGuire, Theodore F. Robles, and Ronald Glaser, "Psychoneuroimmunology: Psychological Influences on Immune Function and Health," *Journal of Consulting and Clinical Psychology* 70, no. 3 (2002): 537-547.

[35] Dareen Blakeborough, ""Old People are Useless": Representations of Aging on The Simpsons," *Canadian Journal on Aging/La Revue Canadienne du Vieillissement* 27, no. 1 (2008): 57-67. E. Shien Chang, Sneha Kannoth, Samantha Levy, Shi-Yi Wang, John E. Lee, and Becca R. Levy, "Global Reach of Ageism on Older Persons' Health: A Systematic Review," *PloS one* 15, no. 1 (2020): e0220857. World Health Organization, *Global Report on Ageism* (World Health Organization, 2021). Accessed February 7, 2023 at https://apps.who.int/iris/bitstream/handle/10665/340208/9789240016866-eng.pdf.

[36] For example, see works by, Rosalia Baena, "Recognition and Empathy in Illness and Disability Memoirs. Christina Middlebrook's Seeing the Crab and Harriet McBryde Johnson's Too Late to Die Young," *Diegesis* 6, no. 2 (2017). Sayantani DasGupta and Rita Charon, "Personal Illness Narratives: Using Reflective Writing to Teach Empathy," *Academic Medicine* 79, no. 4 (2004): 351-356. Andreas M. Krafft, "Stress-Related Growth," In *Our Hopes, Our Future: Insights from the Hope Barometer* (Berlin: Springer Berlin Heidelberg, 2023): 81-87. Shaunna Siler, Kelly Arora, Katherine Doyon, and Stacy M. Fischer, "Spirituality and The Illness Experience: Perspectives of African American Older Adults," *American Journal of Hospice and Palliative Medicine®* 38, no. 6 (2021): 618-625.

[37] Amy L. Ai, "Daoist Spirituality and Philosophy: Implications for Holistic Health, Aging, and Longevity," *Holistic Approaches to Health Aging: Complementary and Alternative Medicine for Older Adults* (New York, NY: Springer, 2006): 149-160. Kristin J. Homan, "Self-compassion and Psychological Well-being in Older Adults," *Journal of Adult Development* 23 (2016): 111-119. Hannah Nguyen, Jung-Ah Lee, Dara H. Sorkin, and Lisa Gibbs, ""Living Happily Despite Having an Illness": Perceptions of Healthy Aging among Korean American, Vietnamese American, and Latino Older Adults," *Applied Nursing Research* 48 (2019): 30-36. Carol D. Ryff, "Psychological Well-Being in Adult Life," *Current Directions in Psychological Science* 4, no. 4 (1995): 99-104. Bram Vanhoutte, "The Multidimensional Structure of Subjective Well-being in Later Life," *Journal of Population Ageing* 7, no. 1 (2014): 1-20.

[38] Kryss McKenna, Kieran Broome, and Jacki Liddle, "What Older People Do: Time Use and Exploring the Link Between Role Participation and Life Satisfaction in People Aged 65 Years and Over," *Australian Occupational Therapy Journal* 54, no. 4 (2007): 273-284. Janine L. Wiles, Kirsty Wild, Ngaire Kerse, and Ruth E.S. Allen, "Resilience From the Point of View of Older People: There's Still Life Beyond a Funny Knee'," *Social Science & Medicine* 74, no. 3 (2012): 416-424. Furthermore, noting that aspects of one's identity and self-agency are still retained even when dementia occurs (see reports by Geraldine Boyle, "Recognising the Agency of People with Dementia," *Disability & Society* 29, no. 7 (2014): 1130-1144; and, Juliette Brown, "Self and Identity Over time: Dementia," *Journal of Evaluation in Clinical Practice 23*, no. 5 (2017): 1006-1012), we also find within various cultural settings an interpretation of cognitive decline to be a normal part of the circle-of-life, or an aspect of one's return to the time of childhood, or an expression of the person's communications with and insight into the supernatural world (see, Gabriele Cipriani and Gemma Borin, "Understanding Dementia in the Sociocultural Context: A Review," *International Journal of Social Psychiatry* 61, no. 2 (2015): 198-204. J. Neil Henderson and L. Carson Henderson, "Cultural Construction of Disease: A "Supernormal" Construct of Dementia in an American Indian Tribe," *Journal of Cross-Cultural Gerontology* 17 (2002): 197-212. Kristen Jacklin and Jennifer Qualitative Evidence Synthesis," *Canadian Journal on Aging/La Revue Canadienne du Vieillissement* 39, no. 2 (2020): 220-234. Emma L. Wolverson, Christopher Clarke, and E. D. Moniz-Cook, "Living Positively with Dementia: A Systematic Review and Synthesis of the Qualitative Literature," *Aging & Mental Health* 20, no. 7 (2016): 676-699). Thus despite cognitive impairment or other functional loss, each person is still important, and their life is imbued with a special meaning and purpose. This whole person characterization alludes to the psychic reality of our existential concerns in later life.

[39] See for example research by, William J. Strawbridge, Sarah J. Shema, Richard D. Cohen, Robert E. Roberts, and George A. Kaplan, "Religiosity Buffers Effects of Some Stressors on Depression but Exacerbates Others," *The Journals of Gerontology Series B: Psychological Sciences and Social Sciences* 53, no. 3 (1998): S118-S126. Joel Savishinsky, "The Passions of Maturity: Morality and Creativity in Later Life," *Journal of Cross-Cultural Gerontology* 16 (2001): 41-55. Karen M. Van Leeuwen et al., *PloS one* 14, no. 3 (2019): e0213263. Paul Wink and Michelle Dillon, "Religiousness, Spirituality, and Psychosocial Functioning in Late Adulthood: Findings from a Longitudinal Study," *Psychology and Aging* 18, no. 4 (2003): 916-924.

[40] Gene D. Cohen, "New Theories and Research Findings on the Positive Influence of Music and Art on Health with Ageing," *Arts & Health* 1, no. 1 (2009): 48-62. Daisy Fancourt and Andrew Steptoe, "The Art of Life and Death: 14 Year Follow-up Analyses of Associations Between Arts Engagement and Mortality in the English Longitudinal Study of Ageing," *British Medical Journal,* 367 (2019): l6377. Colin J. Greaves and Lou Farbus, "Effects of Creative and Social Activity on the Health and Well-being of Socially Isolated Older People: Outcomes from a Multi-method Observational Study," *The Journal of the Royal Society for the Promotion of Health* 126, no. 3 (2006): 134-142. Fidel Molina-Luque, Ieva Stončikaitė, Teresa Torres-González, and Paquita Sanvicen-Torné, "Profiguration, "Active Ageing, and Creativity: Keys for Quality of Life and Overcoming Ageism," *International Journal of Environmental Research and Public Health* 19, no. 3 (2022): 1564. Senhu Wang, Hei Wan Mak, and Daisy Fancourt, "Arts, Mental Distress, Mental Health Functioning & Life Satisfaction: Fixed-effects Analyses of a Nationally-Representative Panel Study." *BMC Public Health* 20 (2020): 1-9.

[41] Kayleigh A. Abbott, Matthew J. Shanahan, and Richard WJ Neufeld, "Artistic Tasks Outperform Nonartistic Tasks for Stress Reduction," *Art Therapy* 30, no. 2 (2013): 71-78.

[42] Hon Keung Yeun, Kris Mueller, Ellise Mayor, and Andres Azuero, "Impact of Participation in a Theatre Programme on Quality of Life Among Older Adults with Chronic Conditions: A Pilot Study," *Occupational Therapy International* 18, no. 4 (2011): 201-208.

[43] Myoung Ae Choe and Heber Lou, "A Study of Dance Movement Training on the Wellness of Young Women," *The Journal of Nurses Academic Society* 25, no. 3 (1995): 538-548.

[44] Krista Curl, "Assessing Stress Reduction as a Function of Artistic Creation and Cognitive Focus," *Art Therapy* 25, no. 4 (2008): 164-169.

[45] Rotem Perac and Arnaud Wisman, "Can Creativity Beat Death? A Review and Evidence on the Existential Anxiety Buffering Functions of Creative Achievement," *The Journal of Creative Behavior* 53, no. 2 (2019): 193-210.

[46] Dean D. VonDras, "Rick Belcher and Meryl Shechter Life Story Interviews with Dean D. VonDras," September, 2020—May, 2021.

[47] Mary E. Fischer, Karen J. Cruickshanks, Barbara E.K. Klein, Ronald Klein, Carla R. Schubert, and Terry L. Wiley, "Multiple Sensory Impairment and Quality of Life," *Ophthalmic Epidemiology* 16:6 (2009): 346-353.

[48] See reports by, Raffaella Boi, Luca Racca, Antonio Cavallero, Veronica Carpaneto, Matteo Racca, Francesca Dall'Acqua, Michele Ricchetti, Alida Santelli, and Patrizio Odetti, "Hearing Loss and Depressive Symptoms in Elderly Patients," *Geriatrics & Gerontology International* 12:3 (2012): 440-445. Louise Hickson, Carly Meyer, Karen Lovelock, Michelle Lampert, and Asad Khan, "Factors Associated with Success with Hearing Aids in Older Adults," *International Journal of Audiology* 53:sup1 (2014): S18-S27.

[49] See reports by, Rokiah Omar and Jalan Raja Muda Abdul Aziz, "Low Vision Rehabilitation Can Improve Quality of Life," *Jurnal Kebajikan Masyarakat* 36 (2010): 99-110. Giulia Renieri, Susanne Pitz, Norbert Pfeiffer, Manfred E. Beutel, and Rüdiger Zwerenz, "Changes in Quality of Life in Visually Impaired Patients After Low-Vision Rehabilitation," *International Journal of Rehabilitation Research* 36:1 (2013): 48-55.

[50] See the reports by, Mark Brennan and Scott J. Bally, "Psychosocial Adaptations to Dual Sensory Loss in Middle and Late Adulthood," *Trends in Amplification* 11:4 (2007): 281-300. Chyrisse Heine and C. J. Browning, "Communication and Psychosocial Consequences of Sensory Loss in Older Adults: Overview and Rehabilitation Directions," *Disability and Rehabilitation* 24:15 (2002): 763-773.

[51] Professor Mitch Wadley, *Little Red Riding Hood (Featuring the Paper Bag)* (St. Louis MO: Mitchell Wadley, 1983); used with permission.

[52] Professor Mitch Wadley, "Mitch Wadley Life Story Interview with Dean D. VonDras" (August 16, 2020; May, 24, 2021).

[53] Find and listen to Professor Mitch Wadley's *Extra Terrestrial Fonk* album at https://www.youtube.com/watch?v=w1HVk4oP2Ps&list=OLAK5uy_nD7fyk5P TM3wuFYfh9IpH-BwSqD_fIkZ8.

[54] Scott F. Madey and Dean D. VonDras, *Music, Wellness, and Aging: Defining, Directing, and Celebrating Life* (New York, NY: Cambridge University Press, 2021).

[55] Jim Weatherhead, "Personal Communication to Dean D. VonDras" (July 4, 2020). Also see, Jim Weatherhead, "Blessed Man's Journey," *The Faces of Ankylosing Spondylitis*, April 17, 2019. Accessed February 14, 2023, at https://thefacesofankylosingspondylitis.com/an-as-life-a-blessed-mans-journey/

[56] Jim Weatherhead (July 4, 2020); used with permission.

CHAPTER SEVEN – MOVE DOWNSTAGE LEFT — THEN WALK TO CENTER

[1] Henry David Thoreau, *Walking* (In the public domain, Concord, 1862).

[2] When we begin an exercise routine, even regular walking, we should always listen to our bodies and be careful not to "over-do-it." Keep in mind that strenuous physical activity can be over-taxing for anyone, at any age. So, consult with your physician prior to starting a new routine of exercise or walking, and perhaps also recruit a friend to accompany you, so as to proceed in the safest manner given one's particular health or medical condition.

[3] Stephanie Studenski, Subashan Perera, Kushang Patel, Caterina Rosano, Kimberly Faulkner, Marco Inzitari, Jennifer Brach et al., "Gait Speed and Survival in Older Adults," *Journal of the American Medical Association* 305:1 (2011): 50-58.

[4] Thomas N. Robinson, Daniel S. Wu, Angela Sauaia, Christina L. Dunn, Jennifer E. Stevens-Lapsley, Marc Moss, Greg V. Stiegmann, Csaba Gajdos, Joseph C. Cleveland Jr, and Sharon K. Inouye, "Slower Walking Speed Forecasts Increased Postoperative Morbidity and One-Year Mortality Across Surgical Specialties," *Annals of Surgery* 258, no. 4 (2013): 582.

[5] Benjumin Hsu, Dafna Merom, Fiona M. Blyth, Vasi Naganathan, Vasant Hirani, David G. Le Couteur, Markus J. Seibel, Louise M. Waite, David J. Handelsman, and Robert G. Cumming, "Total Physical Activity, Exercise Intensity, and Walking Speed as Predictors of All-Cause and Cause-Specific Mortality Over 7 Years in Older Men: The Concord Health and Aging in Men Project," *Journal of the American Medical Directors Association* 19, no. 3 (2018): 216-222.

[6] See reports by Katrine Karmisholt, and Peter C. Gøtzsche, "Physical Activity for Secondary Prevention of Disease: Systematic Reviews of Randomised Clinical Trials," *Danish Medical Bulletin* 52, no. 2 (2005): 90-94; Alpa V. Patel, Janet S. Hildebrand, Corinne R. Leach, Peter T. Campbell, Colleen Doyle, Kerem Shuval, Ying Wang, and Susan M. Gapstur. "Walking in Relation to Mortality in a Large Prospective Cohort of Older US Adults," *American Journal of Preventive Medicine* 54, no. 1 (2018): 10-19; and, Wenjing Zhao, Shigekazu Ukawa, Takashi Kawamura, Kenji Wakai, Masahiko Ando, Kazuyo Tsushita, and Akiko Tamakoshi, "Health Benefits of Daily Walking on Mortality Among Younger-Elderly Men with or Without Major Critical Diseases in the New Integrated Suburban Seniority Investigation Project: A Prospective Cohort Study," *Journal of Epidemiology* 25, no. 10 (2015): 609-616.

[7] Eric B. Larson, L. I. Wang, James D. Bowen, Wayne C. McCormick, Linda Teri, Paul Crane, and Walter Kukull, "Exercise is Associated with Reduced Risk for Incident Dementia Among Persons 65 Years of Age and Older," *Annals of Internal Medicine* 144, no. 2 (2006): 73-81.

[8] Robert D. Abbott, Lon R. White, G. Webster Ross, Kamal H. Masaki, J. David Curb, and Helen Petrovitch, "Walking and Dementia in Physically Capable Elderly Men," *JAMA* 292, no. 12 (2004): 1447-1453.

[9] Yohko Maki, Chiakie Ura, Tomaharu Yamaguchi, Tasuhiko Murai, Mikie Isahai, et al., "Effects of Intervention Using a Community-Based Walking Program for Prevention of Mental Decline: A Randomized Control Trial," *Journal of the American Geriatrics Society* 60, Issue 3 (2012): 505-510.

[10] Diana E. Bowler, Lisette M. Buyung-Ali, Teri M. Knight, and Andrew S. Pullin, "A Systematic Review of Evidence for the Added Benefits to Health of Exposure to Natural Environments," *BMC Public Health* 10, no. 1 (2010): 1-10. Jo Thompson Coon, Kate Boddy, Ken Stein, Rebecca Whear, Joanne Barton, and Michael H. Depledge, "Does Participating in Physical Activity in Outdoor Natural Environments Have a Greater Effect on Physical and Mental Wellbeing than Physical Activity Indoors? A Systematic Review," *Environmental Science & Technology* 45, no. 5 (2011): 1761-1772.

11 Hayley Christian, Adrian Bauman, Jacqueline N. Epping, Glenn N. Levine, Gavin McCormack, Ryan E. Rhodes, Elizabeth Richards, Melanie Rock, and Carri Westgarth, "Encouraging Dog Walking for Health Promotion and Disease Prevention," *American Journal of Life Style Medicine* 12, no. 3 (2018): 233-243.

12 For example, Bill Bryson, *A Walk in the Woods: Rediscovering America on the Appalachian Trail* (New York: Random House, 1998); and, Robert Rubin, *On the Beaten Path: An Appalachian Pilgrimage* (Lanham, Maryland: Rowman & Littlefield, 2009).

13 See the works of Adam Berg, ""To conquer Myself": The New Strenuosity and The Emergence of "Thru-Hiking" on the Appalachian Trail in the 1970s," *Journal of Sport History* 42, no. 1 (2015): 1-19; and, Susan Power Bratton, *The Spirit of the Appalachian Trail: Community, Environment, and Belief* (Knoxville, Tennessee: University of Tennessee Press, 2012).

14 Appalachian Trail Conservancy, "The Adventure of a Lifetime: 2000 Milers," n.d. Accessed on February 4, 2022 at https://appalachiantrail.org/explore/hike-the-a-t/thru-hiking/2000-milers/

15 Nicola Rodriguez, *Sail Away: How to Escape the Rat Race and Live the Dream (Vol. 2).* (Leamington Spa, UK: Fernhurst Books Limited, 2019).

16 See for example, Christian Williams, *Philosophy of Sailing: Offshore in Search of the Universe* (Los Angeles, CA: East Wind Press, 2018).

17 U.S. Sailing Organization, "U.S. Sailing Membership Demographics;" accessed on the world-wide web February 7, 2022 at https://www.ussailing.org/wp-content/uploads/2018/01/Demographics2010.pdf.

18 U.S. Sailing Organization, "Singlehanded Transpac 2018: The Adventure of a Lifetime," n.d. accessed on February 7, 2022 at http://sfbaysss.org/shtp2018/racers/

19 Daniel Wade, "Am I Too Old for Sailing?" *Life of Sailing,* October 1, 2021; accessed February 7, 2022 on the world-wide web at https://www.lifeofsailing.com/post/am-i-too-old-for-sailing; Quantum Sails, "Advice From a 91-Year-old Sailor: You've Got to Keep on Keeping On," *QuantumSails,* October 15, 2015; access February 9, 2022 at https://www.quantumsails.com/en/resources-and-expertise/articles/advice-from-a-91-year-old-sailor-you-ve-got-to-ke

20 DeepSailing, "Sailing a Catamaran: Everything You Need to Know" n.d. Accessed February 7, 2022 at https://www.deepsailing.com/blog/sailing-a-catamaran

21 Robert G. Santee, "Robert G. Santee Interview with Dean D. VonDras." May 26, 2021. For examples of exercises mentioned see the YouTube video, "8 Changes Circle Waling with Wang Shangzie and Zhang Xiu 11-29-14." Accessed February 2, 2022, at https://youtu.be/gQodatOKv-c

[22] For example, see reports by Kelsey T. Laird, Pattharee Paholpak, Michael Roman, Berna Rahi, and Helen Lavretsky, "Mind-Body Therapies for Late-Life Mental and Cognitive health," *Current Psychiatry Reports* 20, no. 1 (2018): 1-12. Albert Yeung, Jessie S.M. Chan, Joey C. Cheung, and Liye Zou, "Qigong and Tai-Chi for Mood Regulation," *Focus* 16, no. 1 (2018): 40-47.

[23] Peter M. Wayne, Jeffrey M. Hausdorff, Matthew Lough, Brian J. Gow, Lewis Lipsitz, Vera Novak, Eric A. Macklin, Chung-Kang Peng, and Brad Manor, "Tai Chi Training May Reduce Dual Task Gait Variability, A Potential Mediator of Fall Risk, In Healthy Older Adults: Cross-Sectional and Randomized Trial Studies," *Frontiers in Human Neuroscience* 9 (2015): 332.

[24] Hector W.H. Tsang, William W.N. Tsang, Alice Y.M. Jones, Kelvin M.T. Fung, Alan H.L. Chan, Edward P. Chan, and Doreen W.H. Au, "Psycho-Physical and Neurophysiological Effects of Qigong on Depressed Elders with Chronic Illness," *Aging & Mental Health* 17, no. 3 (2013): 336-348.

[25] See reports by Peter M. Wayne, Jacquelyn N. Walsh, Ruth E. Taylor-Piliae, Rebecca E. Wells, Kathryn V. Papp, Nancy J. Donovan, and Gloria Y. Yeh, "Effect Of Tai Chi On Cognitive Performance In Older Adults: Systematic Review and Meta-Analysis," *Journal of the American Geriatrics Society* 62, no. 1 (2014): 25-39; and, Jingjing Yang, Lulu Zhang, Qianyun Tang, Fengling Wang, Yu Li, Hua Peng, and Shuhong Wang, "Tai Chi Is Effective In Delaying Cognitive Decline in Older Adults with Mild Cognitive Impairment: Evidence From a Systematic Review and Meta-Analysis," *Evidence-Based Complementary and Alternative Medicine* 2020 (2020).

[26] Wuwei refers to the Daoist practice of not taking action that is not a part of the universe's natural course; Ziran refers to the Daoist concept of being natural and spontaneous, in being as it is. For more on this topic see the following works: Robert G. Santee, *It's Time for a Change: A Therapeutic Lifestyle Approach to Health and Well-Being* (San Diego, CA: Cognella Academic Publishing, 2020); UNESCO, "Taijiqua, China: Inscribed in 2020 (15.COM) on the Representative List of the Intangible Cultural Heritage of Humanity," n.d. Accessed on February 2, 2022, at https://ich.unesco.org/en/RL/taijiquan-00424; and Dang Xiaofei, "Taijiquan: Heritage for Humanity," *China Today*, March 1, 2021. Accessed on the world-wide web on February 2, 2022, at http://www.chinatoday.com.cn/ctenglish/2018/cs/202103/t20210301_800237528.html.

[27] Ruth E. Taylor-Piliae, "Tai Chi as an Adjunct to Cardiac Rehabilitation Exercise Training," *Journal of Cardiopulmonary Rehabilitation and Prevention* 23, no. 2 (2003): 90-96.

[28] Romy Lauche, Wenbo Peng, Caleb Ferguson, Holger Cramer, Jane Frawley, Jon Adams, and David Sibbritt, "Efficacy of Tai Chi and Qigong for the Prevention of Stroke and Stroke Risk Factors: A Systematic Review with Meta-Analysis," *Medicine* 96, no. 45 (2017).

29 Joseph F Audette, Young Soo Jin, Renee Newcomer, Lauren Stein, Gillian Duncan, and Walter R. Frontera, "Tai Chi Versus Brisk Walking in Elderly Women," *Age and Ageing* 35, no. 4 (2006): 388-393.

30 Chunlin Yue, Yanjie Zhang, Mei Jian, Fabian Herold, Qian Yu, Patrick Mueller, Jingyuan Lin et al., "Differential Effects of Tai Chi Chuan (Motor-Cognitive Training) and Walking on Brain Networks: A Resting-State fMRI Study in Chinese Women Aged 60," In *Healthcare*, vol. 8, no. 1, p. 67. Multidisciplinary Digital Publishing Institute, 2020.

31 See, for example, works by, Cook, Langdon Cook, *The Mushroom Hunters: On the Trail of an Underground America* (New York: Ballantine Books, 2013). Euell Gibbons, *Stalking the Wild Asparagus* (New York: David McKay Company,1962). Euell Gibbons, *Stalking the Good Life: My Love Affair with Nature* (New York: David McKay, 1971).

32 Ed Brooker and Marion Joppe, "A Critical Review of Camping Research and Direction for Future Studies," *Journal of Vacation Marketing* 20, no. 4 (2014): 335-351.

33 Deborah Sugerman, "Motivations of Older Adults to Participate in Outdoor Adventure Experiences," *Journal of Adventure Education & Outdoor Learning* 1, no. 2 (2001): 21-33.

34 Brittney Grant, Susan MacDermott, Becki Cohill, and Karen Park, "Increasing Engagement in the Occupation of Camping for Older Adults," Poster Presented at the *Virtual OTD Capstone Symposium, University of St Augustine for Health Sciences* (December 11, 2020).

35 Dan Buettner and Sam Skemp, "Blue Zones: Lessons from the World's Longest Lived," *American Journal of Lifestyle Medicine* 10, no. 5 (2016): 318-321.

36 Jessica Finlay, Thea Franke, Heather McKay, and Joanie Sims-Gould, "Therapeutic Landscapes and Wellbeing in Later Life: Impacts of Blue and Green Spaces for Older Adults," *Health & Place* 34 (2015): 97-106.

37 See respectively works by, Eric Jaffe, "This Side of Paradise," *APS Observer* 23 (2010): 11-15; and, Jo Barton and Jules Pretty, "What is the Best Dose of Nature and Green Exercise for Improving Mental Health? A Multi-Study Analysis," *Environmental Science & Technology* 44, no. 10 (2010): 3947-3955.

38 Margarita Triguero-Mas, David Donaire-Gonzalez, Edmund Seto, Antònia Valentín, David Martínez, Graham Smith, Gemma Hurst et al., "Natural Outdoor Environments and Mental Health: Stress as a Possible Mechanism," *Environmental Research* 159 (2017): 629-638.

39 Peter Aspinall, Panagiotis Mavros, Richard Coyne, and Jenny Roe, "The Urban Brain: Analysing Outdoor Physical Activity with Mobile EEG," *British Journal of Sports Medicine* 49, no. 4 (2015): 272-276.

40 Ruth McCaffrey and Susan B. Raddock, "The Effect of a Reflective Garden Walking Program," *Journal of Therapeutic Horticulture* 23, no. 1 (2013): 23-34.

41 Ruth McCaffrey and Patricia Liehr, "The Effect of Reflective Garden Walking on Adults with Increased Levels of Psychological Stress," *Journal of Holistic Nursing* 34, no. 2 (2016): 177-184.

[42] Carina S. Bichler, Martin Niedermeier, Katharina Hüfner, Matyas Galffy, Barbara Sperner-Unterweger, and Martin Kopp, "Affective Responses to Both Climbing and Nordic Walking Exercise are Associated with Intermediate-Term Increases in Physical Activity in Patients with Anxiety and Posttraumatic Stress Disorder - A Randomized Longitudinal Controlled Clinical Plot Trial," *Frontiers in Psychiatry* 13 (2022). Martin Niedermeier, Jürgen Einwanger, Arnulf Hartl, and Martin Kopp, "Affective Responses in Mountain Hiking—A Randomized Crossover Trial Focusing on Differences Between Indoor and Outdoor Activity" *PLoS one* 12, no. 5 (2017): e0177719.

[43] Jennifer Walsh and Beth McGroarty, "Prescribing Nature: There is Enough Science About the Health Benefits of Nature to Get the Attention of the Medical Profession. Nature as Medicine. Just Don't Tell Big Pharma," *2019 Wellness Trends, from the Global Wellness Summit.* Accessed March 12, 2023 at https://www.globalwellnesssummit.com/2019-global-wellness-trends/prescribing-nature/

[44] Monty Don, *The Jewel Garden: A Story of Despair and Redemption* (London, United Kingdom: Two Roads, 2004).

[45] Donna Wang and Allen Glicksman, ""Being grounded": Benefits of Gardening for Older Adults in Low-Income Housing," *Journal of Housing for the Elderly* 27, no. 1-2 (2013): 89-104.

[46] Sean O. Nicholas, Anh T. Giang, and Philip L.K. Yap, "The Effectiveness of Horticultural Therapy on Older Adults: A Systematic Review," *Journal of the American Medical Directors Association* 20, no. 10 (2019): 1351-e1.

[47] Christine Milligan, Anthony Gatrell, and Amanda Bingley, "'Cultivating Health': Therapeutic Landscapes and Older People in Northern England," *Social Science & Medicine* 58, no. 9 (2004): 1781-1793

[48] Kyung-Hee Kim and Sin-Ae Park, "Horticultural Therapy Program for Middle-Aged Women's Depression, Anxiety, and Self-identify," *Complementary Therapies in Medicine* 39 (2018): 154-159.

[49] Claudia K.Y. Lai, Rick Y.C. Kwan, Shirley K.L. Lo, Connie Y.Y. Fung, Jordan K.H. Lau, and M. Y. Mimi, "Effects of Horticulture on Frail and Prefrail Nursing Home Residents: A Randomized Controlled Trial," *Journal of the American Medical Directors Association* 19, no. 8 (2018): 696-702.

[50] Thomas A. Cornille, Glenn E. Rohrer, and Jean G. Mosier, "Horticultural Therapy in Substance Abuse Treatment," *Journal of Therapeutic Horticulture* (1987): 3-7; F. Ferrini, "Horticultural Therapy and Its Effect on People's Health," *Horticultural Therapy and Its Effect on People's Health* (2003): 1000-1011.

[51] James Hollis, *Living an Examined Life: Wisdom for the Second Half of the Journey* (Boulder, Colorado: Sounds True, 2018).

[52] Weilin Chen, Hongmei Ma, Xiao Wang, and Jiaojiao Chen, "Effects of a Death Education Intervention for Older People with Chronic Disease and Family Caregivers: A Quasi-Experimental Study," *Asian Nursing Research* 14, no. 4 (2020): 257-266. Julia T. Robinson and Amy B. Murphy-Nugen, "It Makes You Keep Trying: Life Review Writing for Older Adults," *Journal of Gerontological Social Work* 61, no. 2 (2018): 171-192. Shuji Tsuda, Mami Jinno, and Satoko Hotta, "Exploring the Meaning of Journal Writing in People Living with Dementia: A Qualitative Study," *Psychogeriatrics* 22, no. 5 (2022): 699-706.

[53] Chih-Hsiang Yang, and David E. Conroy, "Feasibility of an Outdoor Mindful Walking Program for Reducing Negative Affect in Older Adults," *Journal of Aging and Physical Activity* 27, no. 1 (2019): 18-27.

[54] Martin Mau, Dorthe S. Nielsen, Ida Skytte Jakobsen, Søren H. Klausen, and Kirsten K. Roessler, "Mental Movements: How Long-Distance Walking Influences Reflection Processes Among Middle-Age and Older Adults," *Scandinavian Journal of Psychology* 62, no. 3 (2021): 365-373.

[55] Dustin W. Davis, "A Literature Review on the Physiological and Psychological Effects of Labyrinth Walking," *International Journal of Yogic, Human Movement and Sports Sciences* 6, no. 1 (2021): 167-175.

CHAPTER EIGHT – BUT THAT IS NOT HOW THE STORY ENDS: A RESPONSE TO THE COVID-19 PANDEMIC AND MOVING BEYOND

[1] World Health Organization, "The World Health Organization Coronavirus Disease (Covid-19) Dashboard." The World Health Organization Coronavirus Disease (Covid-19). Accessed December 30, 2022 at https://covid19.who.int.

[2] Centers for Disease Control and Prevention, "COVID-19 Vaccines & Boosters." Accessed March 20, 2023 at https://www.cdc.gov/coronavirus/2019-ncov/index.html.

[3] Hans C. Andersen, *What the Moon Saw: And Other Tales*, H. W. Dulcken, trans. (In the public domain, 1866): 39.

[4] Jem Asward, "Sofar Sounds, Host of Intimate and Secret Concerts, Returns form Pandemic Bigger Than Ever," *Variety*, June 13, 2023. Accessed July 3, 2023 at https://variety.com/2023/music/news/sofar-sounds-returns-pandemic-1235641488/. Missy Durant, "The World Changed During the Pandemic. So Did We. Now Flexibility in Where and How Work Gets Done is Key," *StarTribune*, June 18, 2023. Accessed July 3, 2023 at https://www.startribune.com/the-world-changed-during-the-pandemic-so-did-we/600283614/.

[5] Norman Lebrecht, "A Full Assessment of the Covid Risk of Playing Wind Instruments," *SlippedDisc*, June 11, 2020. Accessed March 20, 2023 at https://slippedisc.com/2020/06/a-full-assessment-of-the-covid-risk-of-playing-wind-instruments/

6 For example, Tehya Stockman, Shengwei Zhu, Abhishek Kumar, Lingzhe Wang, Sameer Patel, James Weaver, Mark Spede et al., "Measurements and Simulations of Aerosol Released While Singing and Playing Wind Instruments," *ACS Environmental Au* 1, no. 1 (2021): 71-84.

7 Ruichen He, Linyue Gao, Maximillian Trifonov, and Jiarong Hong, "Aerosol Generation From Different Wind Instruments," *Journal of Aerosol Science* 151 (September 16, 2020): 1-11.

8 Dylan Vance, Priyanka Shah, and Robert T. Sataloff, "Covid 19: Impact on the Musician and Returning to Singing; A Literature Review," *Journal of Voice* 37, no. 2 (2023): 292-e1.

9 Advisory from the AMTA Covid-19 Task Force, "Does Singing, Speech, and/or Playing a Wind/Blow Instrument Amplify Viral Spread?" (April 23, 2020). Accessed April 12, 2021 at https://www.musictherapy.org/advisory_from_the_amta_covid19_task_force/

10 Rehearsal Protocols of The Carlisle Town Band, Carlisle, PA (used with permission, accessed March,14, 2021).

11 D. Vance et al, *Journal of Voice* 37, no. 2 (2023): 292-e1.

12 Felicia K. Youngblood, Joanna Bosse, and Cameron T. Whitley, "How Can I Keep From Singing? The Effect of Covid-19 on the Emotional Wellbeing of Community Singers During Early Stage Lockdown in the United States," *International Journal of Community Music* 14, no. 2-3 (2021): 205-221.

13 Noah R. Fram, Visda Goudarzi, Hiroko Terasawa, and Jonathan Berger, "Collaborating in Isolation: Assessing the Effects of the Covid-19 Pandemic on Patterns of Collaborative Behavior Among Working Musicians," *Frontiers in Psychology*, 12, 674246.

14 Christine Carter, "Why the Progress You Make in the Practice Room Seems to Disappear Overnight—Part 1," *BulletProofMusician* (n.d.). Accessed April 25, 2021 at https://bulletproofmusician.com/why-the-progress-in-the-practice-room-seems-to-disappear-overnight/

15 Dean D. VonDras and Scott F. Madey, "The Attainment of Important Health Goals Throughout Adulthood: An Integration of the Theory of Planned Behavior and Aspects of Social Support," *International Journal of Aging and Human Development* 59, no. 3 (2004), pp. 205–234.

16 Dean D. VonDras and Scott F. Madey, "Perceived Spousal Support and Attainment of Health Goals in Later Life," *International Journal of Personality Research* 8, no. 1 (2013), pp. 1–16.

17 Mary Louise Kelly (Host). "Yo-Yo Ma, A Life Led With Bach, Tiny Desk Concert," *WITF*, https://www.npr.org/transcripts/639571356), (accessed March 14, 2021).

18 Susan Folkman, Richard S. Lazarus, Christine Dunkel-Schetter, Anita DeLongis, and Rand J. Gruen, "Dynamics of a Stressful Encounter: Cognitive Appraisal, Coping, and Encounter Outcomes," *Journal of Personality and Social Psychology* 505 (1986): 992-1003.

19 VonDras and Madey, 205-234.

[20] Teresia Lesiuk, "The Development of a Mindfulness-Based Music Therapy (MBMT) Program for Women Receiving Adjuvant Chemotherapy for Breast Cancer," *Healthcare* 4 (2014), pp. 1–14.

[21] Dean D. VonDras, "Interview with Br. A. Brian Zampier" (September, 2021).

[22] Centers for Disease Control and Prevention (CDC), "Interim Public Health Recommendations for Fully Vaccinated People." Access April 26, 2021 at https://www.cdc.gov/coronavirus/2019-ncov/vaccines/fully-vaccinated-guidance.

[23] N. R. Fram et al., *Frontiers in Psychology*, *12*, 674246.

[24] Centers for Disease Control and Prevention, "Stay Up to Date with COVID-19 Vaccines Including Boosters," March 2, 2023. Accessed March 20, 2023 at https://www.cdc.gov/coronavirus/2019-ncov/vaccines/fully-vaccinated-guidance.html

[25] Billboard Staff, "Latin Artists Who Have Shared Their Coronavirus Vaccination Experience," *Billboard*, April 27, 2021. Accessed March 20, 2023 at https://www.billboard.com/articles/columns/latin/9549788/latin-artists-who-got-covid-vaccine/

[26] For example, consider the following articles: Amalia Hasnida, Maarten Olivier Kok, and Elizabeth Pisani, "Challenges in Maintaining Medicine Quality While Aiming for Universal Health Coverage: A Qualitative Analysis from Indonesia," *BMJ Global Health* 6, no. Suppl 3 (2021): e003663. Carol Holtz, ed. *Global Health Care: Issues and Policies* (Jones & Bartlett Publishers, 2013). Chenglin Liu, "Leaving the FDA Behind: Pharmaceutical Outsourcing and Drug Safety," *Tex. Int'l LJ* 48 (2012): 1.

[27] World Health Organization, "The World Health Organization Coronavirus Disease (Covid-19) Dashboard." Accessed March 20, 2023 at https://covid19.who.int.

CHAPTER NINE – THE ART OF RESILIENCE

[1] For example, see works by the following authors: Scott T. Allison, George R. Goethals, Allyson R. Marrinan, Owen M. Parker, Smaragda P. Spyrou, and Madison Stein, "The Metamorphosis of the Hero: Principles, Processes, and Purpose," *Frontiers in Psychology* 10 (2019): 606. Heinz Lichtenstein, "The Dilemma of Human Identity: Notes on Self-Transformation, Self-Objectivation, and Metamorphosis," *Journal of the American Psychoanalytic Association* 11, no. 1 (1963): 173-223. Katherine J. Reynolds and Nyla R. Branscombe, eds., *Psychology of Change: Life Contexts, Experiences, and Identities* (New York, NY: Psychology Press, 2015). Ernest G. Schachtel, *Metamorphosis: On the Conflict of Human Development and the Development of Creativity* (New York, NY: Routledge, 2013).

² See both the early psychoanalytic works by, Sigmund Freud, *The Interpretation of Dreams*, trans. by A. A. Brill (New York, NY: The Macmillan Co., 1913); and, Carl Gustav Jung, *The Undiscovered Self: With Symbols and the Interpretation of Dreams*, Vol. 31 (Princeton, NJ: Princeton University Press, 2012); as well as later interpretations by. Karl Albrecht, *Practical Intelligence: The Art and Science of Common Sense* (New York, NY: Wiley, 2007); Stephen A. Diamond, *Anger, Madness, and the Daimonic: The Psychological Genesis of Violence, Evil, and Creativity* (Albany, NY: SUNY Press, 1996); Joel Weinberger and Valentina Stoycheva, *The Unconscious: Theory, Research, and Clinical Implications* (New York, NY: The Guilford Press, 2019); and Irvin D. Yalom, *Existential Psychotherapy* (New York, NY: Basic Books, 1980).

³ For example, confer the following works: Jack J. Bauer, Joseph R. Schwab, and Dan P. McAdams. "Self-actualizing: Where Ego Development Finally Feels Good?," *The Humanistic Psychologist* 39, no. 2 (2011): 121-136; Jeni L. Burnette, Joseph Billingsley, George C. Banks, Laura E. Knouse, Crystal L. Hoyt, Jeffrey M. Pollack, and Stefanie Simon, "A Systematic Review and Meta-analysis of Growth Mindset Interventions: For Whom, How, and Why Might Such Interventions Work?," *Psychological Bulletin* 149, no. 3-4 (2023): 174; Jeni L. Burnette, Laura E. Knouse, Dylan T. Vavra, Ernest O'Boyle, and Milan A. Brooks, "Growth Mindsets and Psychological Distress: A Meta-analysis," *Clinical Psychology Review* 77 (2020): 101816; Chaya R. Jain, Daniel K. Apple, and W. Ellis, "What is Self-growth," *International Journal of Process Education* 7, no. 1 (2015): 41-52; Rollo May and Irvin Yalom, "Existential Psychotherapy," In R. J. Corsini and D. Wedding, eds. *Current Psychotherapies* (Itasca, IL: F.E. Peacock Publishers, 1989): 363-402; Dan P. McAdams, Regina L. Logan, and Hollen N. Reischer, "Beyond the Redemptive Self: Narratives of Acceptance in Later Life (and in Other Contexts)," *Journal of Research in Personality* 100 (2022): 104286; Hollen N. Reischer, Laura J. Roth, Jorge A. Villarreal, and Dan P. McAdams, "Self-Transcendence and Life Stories of Humanistic Growth among Late-Midlife Adults," *Journal of Personality* 89, no. 2 (2021): 305-324; and, Piers Worth, ed., *Positive Psychology Across the Lifespan: An Existential Perspective* (New York, NY: Routledge, 2022).

⁴ Scott F. Madey and Dean D. VonDras, *Music, Wellness, and Aging: Defining, Directing, and Celebrating Life* (New York, NY: Cambridge University Press, 2021): 164. We also recognize the complementing phrase and conceptualization of "metamorphosis" as found in works by John R.F. Gladman, "Personal Growth and Development in Old Age—A Clinician's Perspective," *Age and Ageing* 48, no. 1 (2019): 8-10. Andreas Kruse, "Aging and Personal Growth. Developmental Potentials in Old Age," In M. Schweda, M. Coors, and C. Bozzaro, eds., *Aging and Human Nature: Perspectives from Philosophical, Theological, and Historical Anthropology* (Cham, Switzerland: Springer, 2020): 27-46. Mark Schweda, Michael Coors, and Claudia Bozzaro, eds., *Aging and Human Nature: Perspectives from Philosophical, Theological, and Historical Anthropology* (Cham, Switzerland: Springer, 2020).

[5] Natalie Rogers et al., *Person-Centered & Experiential Psychotherapies* 11, no. 1 (2012): 31-47.

[6] Jennie Cane is the second author's mother-in-law.

[7] Dean D. VonDras, "Rick Belcher and Meryl Shechter Life Story Interviews with Dean D. VonDras," September, 2020—May, 2021.

[8] See, Cancer.Net Editorial Board, "Brain Tumor: Statistics," *Cancer.Net*, March, 2023, Accessed October 4, 2023 at https://www.cancer.net/cancer-types/brain-tumor/statistics; P. A. McKinney, "Brain Tumours: Incidence, Survival, and Aetiology," *Journal of Neurology, Neurosurgery & Psychiatry* 75, no. suppl 2 (2004): ii12-ii17.

[9] "Then & Now: Jon," September 28, 2021, *UW Health Kids*. Accessed January 25, 2022 at *https://www.facebook.com/uwhealthkids/posts/jon-juckem-of-de-pere-wisconsin-was-12-when-he-was-diagnosed-wth-a-life-threate/10161484365262178/*

[10] Marianne Madey is the second author's mother.

[11] Tara Brach, *Radical Acceptance: Embracing Your Life with the Heart of a Buddha* (New York, NY: Bantam Books, 2003): 26.

[12] L. Tornstam, *Journal of Transpersonal Psychology* 43, no. 2 (2011): 166-180.

CHAPTER TEN – VARIOUS SKETCHES AND HUES OF LIFE

[1] Carleton Eldredge Noyes, *The Gate of Appreciation: Studies in the Relation of Art to Life* (in the Public Domain, 1907): 29.

[2] C. E. Noyes (1907): 17.

[3] The Gerontological Society of America, "Creative Approaches to Healthy Aging," 62nd Annual Scientific Meeting, November 18-22, 2009, Atlanta Georgia; Accessed February 15, 2022 at https://www.geron.org/archives/AnnualMeeting/Geron-PreProgram.pdf

[4] Erik Wahl, *Unthink: Rediscover your creative genius* (New York: Crown Business, 2013).

[5] Otto Kallir and Anna Mary Robertson Moses, *Grandma Moses: My Life's History* (New York: Harper & Brothers Publ., 1952).

[6] Hendrik Willem van Loon, *The Life and Times of Rembrandt* (New York: Avon Books, 1957).

[7] Hendrik Willem van Loon, 1957: 249.

[8] Laurie Wilson and Mala Betensky, "Art is the Therapy," in J. A. Rubin, ed., *Approaches to Art Therapy: Theory and Technique (Third Edition)* (New York: Routledge, 2016): 17-32.

[9] Judith Aron Rubin (ed.), *Approaches to Art Therapy: Theory and Technique (Third Edition)* (New York: Routledge, 2016).

[10] See respectively works by, Anita Jensen and Lars Ole Bonde, "The Use of Arts Interventions for Mental Health and Wellbeing in Health Settings," *Perspectives in Public Health* 138, no. 4 (2018): 209-214; and, Stephen Clift, "Creative Arts as a Public Health Resource: Moving from Practice-Based Research to Evidence-Based Practice," *Perspectives in Public Health* 132, no. 3 (2012): 120-127.

[11] Erin Partridge, *Art Therapy with Older Adults: Connected and Empowered* (London: Jessica Kingsley Publishers, 2019).

[12] Adelita G. Cantu, and K. Jill Fleuriet, ""Making the Ordinary More Extraordinary": Exploring Creativity as a Health Promotion Practice Among Older Adults in a Community-Based Professionally Taught Arts Program," *Journal of Holistic Nursing*, 2017, Vol. 36, no. 2 (2107): 123-133.

[13] Berna G. Huebner, *"I Remember Better When I Paint–Art and Alzheimer's: Opening Doors, Making Connections"* (Bethesda, MD: Bethesda Communications Group, 2011).

[14] Janie McMurray, *Creative Ats with Older People* (New York: Routledge, 2018). Amanda Alders Pike, "Art Therapy with Older Adults," In D. E. Gussak and M.L. Rosal (eds.), *The Wiley Handbook of Art Therapy* (Wiley & Sons: West Sussex, UK, 2015): 272-281. Kathleen B. Kahn-Denis, "Art Therapy with Geriatric Dementia Clients," *Art Therapy* 14, no. 3 (1997): 194-199. Tisah Tucknott-Cohen and Crystal Ehresman, "Art Therapy for an Individual with Late Stage Dementia: A Clinical Case Description," *Art Therapy* 33, no. 1 (2016): 41-45.

[15] Rachael Lee, Jonathan Wong, Wong Lit Shoon, Mihir Gandhi, Feng Lei, E. H. Kua, Iris Rawtaer, and Rathi Mahendran, "Art Therapy for the Prevention of Cognitive Decline," *The Arts in Psychotherapy* 64 (2019): 20-25.

[16] Alistair D. Smith, "On the Use of Drawing Tasks in Neuropsychological Assessment," *Neuropsychology* 23, no. 2 (2009): 231.

[17] Jeffrey D. Wammes, Brady R.T. Roberts, and Myra A. Fernandes, "Task Preparation as a Mnemonic: The Benefits of Drawing (and Not Drawing)," *Psychonomic Bulletin & Review* 25, no. 6 (2018): 2365-2372.

[18] Myra A. Fernandes, Jeffrey D. Wammes, and Melissa E. Meade, "The Surprisingly Powerful Influence of Drawing on Memory," *Current Directions in Psychological Science* 27, no. 5 (2018): 302-308. Melissa E. Meade, Jeffrey D. Wammes, and Myra A. Fernandes, "Drawing as an Encoding Tool: Memorial Benefits in Younger and Older Adults," *Experimental Aging Research* 44, no. 5 (2018): 369-396.

[19] Bree Chancellor, Angel Duncan, and Anjan Chatterjee, "Art Therapy for Alzheimer's Disease and Other Dementias," *Journal of Alzheimer's Disease* 39, no. 1 (2014): 1-11.

[20] Jon G. Lyon, "Drawing: Its Value as a Communication Aid for Adults with Aphasia," *Aphasiology* 9, no. 1 (1995): 33-50.

[21] Dana Farias, Christine Davis, and Gregory Harrington, "Drawing: Its Contribution to Naming in Aphasia," *Brain and Language* 97, no. 1 (2006): 53-63.

[22] Cosima Gretton and Dominic H. Ffytche, "Art and the Brain: A View from Dementia," *International Journal of Geriatric Psychiatry* 29, no. 2 (2014): 111-126.

[23] Sarah MacPherson, Michael Bird, Katrina Anderson, Terri Davis, and Annaliese Blair, "An Art Gallery Access Programme for People with Dementia: 'You do it for the moment'," *Aging & Mental Health* 13, no. 5 (2009): 744-752.

[24] Hannah Zeilig, Laura Dickens, and Paul Camic, "The Psychological and Social Impacts of Museum-Based Programmes for People with a Mild-to-Moderate Dementia: A Systematic Review," *International Journal of Ageing and Later Life 16*, no. 2 (2022): 33-72.

[25] Patrick Kabanda, *Work as Art: Links Between Creative Work and Human Development (UNDP,* 2015).

[26] Teresa A. Byington and YaeBin Kim, "Promoting Preschoolers' Emergent Writing," *YC Young Children 72*, no. 5 (2017): 74-82.

[27] Tanner Christensen, *The Creativity Challenge: Design, Experiment, Test, Innovate, Build, Create, Inspire, and Unleash Your Genius* (New York: Simon and Schuster, 2015).

[28] See for example, works by the following: Jackie Andrade, "What Does Doodling Do?," *Applied Cognitive Psychology: The Official Journal of the Society for Applied Research in Memory and Cognition 24*, no. 1 (2010): 100-106. Priyanka Baweja, "Doodling: A Positive Creative Leisure Practice," in, Kone Shintaro, Anju Beniwal, Priyanka Baweja and Karl Spracklen, eds., *Positive Sociology of Leisure* (Cham, Switzerland: Palgrave Macmillan, 2020): 333-349. Milagros I. Rivera Cora, Soledad Gonzales, Matilde Sarmiento, Alejandra Esparza Young, Edith Esparza, Nikolina Madjer, Pinaikini Shankar, Yadmarie Rivera, and Isaac Abulatan, "The Power of a Doodling Brain: Concept Maps as Pathways to Learning," *Education Quarterly Reviews 4*, no. 1 (2021). Tanja Sharpe, *Doodle Your Worries Away: A CBT Doodling Workbook for Children Who Feel Worried Or Anxious* (London: Jessica Kingsley Publishers, 2021).

[29] Deekshita Sundararaman, "Doodle Away: Exploring the Effects of Doodling on Recall Ability of High School Students," *International Journal of Psychological Studies 12*, no. 2 (2020): 31-44.

[30] T. Singh and N. Kashyap, "Does Doodling Effect Performance: Comparison Across Retrieval Strategies," *Psychological Studies 60*, no. 1 (2015): 7-11.

[31] See respectively, research by, Jeffrey D. Wammes, Melissa E. Meade, and Myra A. Fernandes, "The Drawing Effect: Evidence for Reliable and Robust Memory Benefits in Free Recall," *Quarterly Journal of Experimental Psychology 69*, no. 9 (2016): 1752-1776; and, Gianluca Amico and Sabine Schaefer, "No Evidence for Performance Improvements in Episodic Memory Due to Fidgeting, Doodling or a "Neuro-Enhancing" Drink," *Journal of Cognitive Enhancement 4*, no. 1 (2020): 2-11.

[32] Allan B. De Guzman, Hye-Eun Shim, Charmin Kathleen M. Sia, Wilbart Harvey S. Siazon, Mary Joyce Ann P. Sibal, Joanna Brigitte Lorraine C. Siglos, and Francis Marlo C. Simeon, "Ego Integrity of Older People with Physical Disability and Therapeutic Recreation," *Educational Gerontology 37*, no. 4 (2011): 265-291.

[33] Emma Tokolahi, "Case Study: Development of a Drawing-Based Journal to Facilitate Reflective Inquiry," *Reflective Practice 11*, no. 2 (2010): 157-170.

[34] Nantia Koulidou, Jayne Wallace, Miriam Sturdee, and Abigail Durrant. "Drawing on Experiences of Self: Dialogical Sketching," *Proceedings of the 2020 ACM Designing Interactive Systems Conference* (Eindhoven, Netherlands, 2020): 255-267.

[35] Beatriz Martínez Barria, "Peace Treaty: A Dialogue Between the Critical Voice and the Creative Voice," In E. Maisel (ed.), *The Creativity Workbook for Coaches and Creatives* (New York: Routledge, 2020): 55-57.

[36] Theresa C. Maatman, Lana M. Minshew, and Michael T. Braun, "Increase in Sharing of Stressful Situations by Medical Trainees through Drawing Comics," *Journal of Medical Humanities* 43, no. 3 (2022): 467-473.

[37] Jennifer E. Drake, "Examining the Psychological and Psychophysiological Benefits of Drawing Over One month," *Psychology of Aesthetics, Creativity, and the Arts* 13, no. 3 (2019): 338-347.

[38] Nicole Turturro and Jennifer E. Drake, "Does Coloring Reduce Anxiety? Comparing the Psychological and Psychophysiological Benefits of Coloring versus Drawing," *Empirical Studies of the Arts* 40, no. 1 (2022): 3-20.

[39] Brien K. Ashdown, Jamie S. Bodenlos, Kelsey Arroyo, Melanie Patterson, Elena Parkins, and Sarah Burstein, "How Does Coloring Influence Mood, Stress, and Mindfulness?," *Journal of Integrated Social Sciences* 8, no. 1 (2018): 1-21.

[40] Christine Korol and Kimberly Sogge, "The Development of a Contemplative Art Program for Adolescents and Adults: Challenges and Unexpected Benefits," in B. Kirkcaldy, ed., *Psychotherapy, Literature and the Visual and Performing Arts* (Cham, Switzerland: Palgrave Macmillan, 2018): 153-172.

[41] Emma Tokolahi, *Reflective Practice* 11, no. 2 (2010): 157-170.

[42] Dean D. VonDras, from, "Collection of Caricature Essays" (December, 2021). Additional comments from students included the following: "It was fun because it made me think… it opened my mind." – Paige S.; "As I was drawing this caricature, I was in a very positive up-lifting mood." – Dylan J.; "I do not really draw… I did laugh a little, and even though the drawing is serious, it was a stress reliever. Doing something creative is a good outlet for many things." – Faith G.; "I cannot draw… [However,] the inner aspect of myself that the caricature reveals is my belief in God and the reverence I feel during this Holy week… in doing the drawing I discovered that I am thankful." – Joseph L-B.; "This was a fun activity for many reasons. First, I don't remember the last time I drew! It was a creative activity that let my imagination run wild and add whatever I wanted to the picture. It was fun creating an image… [of] hopefully my future. I think this drawing reflects myself not only by my career choice, but it also gives an understanding that I want to make a difference in the world… During this drawing process, I discovered how excited I am for the future." – Kendall R.; "After I completed my entire drawing I remembered how much I enjoyed drawing, stenciling, and painting." – Ashley H.

[43] C. E. Noyes (1907): 29.

44 Pat Allen, "Art Making as a Spiritual Path," in J. A. Rubin, ed., *Approaches to Art Therapy: Theory and Technique (Third Edition)* (New York: Routledge, 2016): 271-285. Michael Franklin, "Contemplative Wisdom Traditions in Art Therapy," in J. A. Rubin, ed., *Approaches to Art Therapy: Theory and Technique (Third Edition)* (New York: Routledge, 2016): 308-330.

45 Dean D. VonDras, "Interview with Br. A. Brian Zampier" (September, 2021).

46 Ekhart Tolle, *Practicing the Power of Now: A Guide to Spiritual Enlightenment* (Hachette: Australia, 2019).

47 Full references for noted works are the following: Frederick Franck, *Art as a Way: A Return to the Spiritual Roots* (Crossroad Publishing Company, 1981); and, Frederick Franck, *The Zen of Seeing: Seeing-Drawing as Meditation* (Vintage, 1973).

48 *The Annual Juried Issue, Letter Arts Review, Volume 32, Number 1*, 2018.

49 Amanda Bustos, "Marianist Brother Spreads Origami Cranes: Flocks for Peace," *Gold & Blue Magazine - St. Mary's University*, March 29, 2018. Accessed November 10, 2022, at https://www.stmarytx.edu/2018/flocks-for-peace/.

50 Takayuki Ishii, *One Thousand Paper Cranes: The Story of Sadako and the Children's Peace Statue* (New York: Laurel Leaf, 2001).

CHAPTER ELEVEN – RENAISSANCE

1 For example, see the following works: John Anthony Burron, *The Ages of Man: A Study in Medieval Writing and Thought* (Oxford, UK: Oxford University Press, 1988). Thorlac Turville-Petre, "The Ages of Man in "The Parlement of the Thre Ages"," *Medium Aevum* 46, no. 1 (1977): 66-76.

2 Peter Laslett, *A Fresh Map of Life: The Emergence of The Third Age* (Cambridge, MA: Harvard University Press, 1991).

3 Robert Browning, *The Compete Poetic and Dramatic Works of Robert Browning, Cambridge Edition*, Horace E. Scudder, ed., (In the public domain, 1895): 384. The poem "Rabbi Ben Ezra" was first published in 1864.

4 P. Laslett (1991): vii.

5 For example, see articles by Valerie A. Braithwaite, "Old Age Stereotypes: Reconciling Contradictions" *Journal of Gerontology* 41, no. 3 (1986): 353-360. Imogen Lyons, "Public Perceptions of Older People and Ageing," *Dublin: National Centre for the Protection of Older People (NCPOP)* (2009): 14. Fred Rothbaum, "Aging and Age Stereotypes." *Social Cognition* 2, no. 2 (1983): 171-184.

6 Thomas R. Cole, *Old Man Country: My Search for Meaning Among the Elders.* (New York: Oxford University Press, 2019).

7 T. R. Cole (2019): 9.

8 T. R. Cole (2019): 11.

[9] Amanda Grenier and Chris Phillipson, "Rethinking Agency in Late Life: Structural and Interpretive Approaches," In J. Baars, J. Dohmen, A. Grenier, and C. Phillipson, eds., *Ageing, Meaning and Social structure. Connecting Critical and Humanistic Gerontology* (Bristol, UK: Policy Press, 2013): 55-79.

[10] For discussion of and reference to these concepts, see respectively the following works: Leni Marshall, *Age Becomes Us: Bodies and Gender in Time* (New York: SUNY Press, 2015): 65; Shawnda Lanting, Margaret Crossley, Debra Morgan, and Allison Cammer, "Aboriginal Experiences of Aging and Dementia in a Context of Sociocultural Change: Qualitative Analysis of Key Informant Group Interviews with Aboriginal Seniors," *Journal of Cross-Cultural Gerontology* 26, no. 1 (2011): 103-117; and, Colette V. Browne, Lana Sue Ka'opua, Lori L. Jervis, Richard Alboroto, and Meredith L. Trockman, "United States Indigenous Populations and Dementia: Is There a Case for Culture-Based Psychosocial Interventions?," *The Gerontologist* 57, no. 6 (2017): 1011-1019.

[11] A. Kruse, *Aging and Human Nature: Perspectives from Philosophical, Theological, and Historical Anthropology* (Cham, Switzerland: Springer, 2020): 27-46. Also, see the works of J. R.F. Gladman, *Age and Ageing* 48, no. 1 (2019): 8-10.

[12] For example, see the following works, Valerie Lander McCarthy and Amanda Bockweg, "The Role of Transcendence in a Holistic View of Successful Aging: A Concept Analysis and Model of Transcendence in Maturation and Aging," *Journal of Holistic Nursing* 31, no. 2 (2013): 84-92. Valerie Lander McCarthy, Lynne A. Hall, Timothy N. Crawford, and Jennifer Connelly, "Facilitating Self-Transcendence: An Intervention to Enhance Well-Being in Late Life," *Western Journal of Nursing Research* 40, no. 6 (2018): 854-873. Valerie Lander McCarthy, Sharon Bowland, Lynne A. Hall, and Jennifer Connelly, "Assessing the Psychoeducational Approach to Transcendence and Health Program: An Intervention to Foster Self-Transcendence and Well-Being in Community-Dwelling Older Adults," *The International Journal of Aging and Human Development* 82, no. 1 (2015): 3-29.

[13] Joanne S. Rupp, *Relevant Last Wishes* ("Permission-to-Use" granted to Dean D. VonDras on 5-18-2021).

[14] Gene Cohen, "Research on Creativity and Aging: The Positive Impact of the Arts on Health and Illness," *Generations* 30, no. 1 (2006): 7-15.

[15] Carl G. Jung, "The Stages of Life," *Volume 8 of the Collected Works of C. G. Jung, second ed.*, (Princeton, NJ: Princeton University Press, 1969): 387-403.

[16] See works by, Bill Cosgrave and Ita Moynihan, "The Midlife Transition," *The Furrow* 46, no. 4 (1995): 210-219. David Gutmann, *The Human Elder in Nature, Culture, and Society (New York, NY: Routledge, 2019). David Gutmann, *Reclaimed Powers: Men and Women in Later Life* (Evanston, IL: Northwestern University Press, 1994). Bernice L. Neugarten, ed. *Middle Age and Aging* (Chicago, IL: University of Chicago Press, 1968). Stephen Palmer and Sheila Panchal, "Modern midlife," in S. Palmer and S. Panchal, eds., *Developmental Coaching* (London: Routledge, 2012): 131-152.

[17] Renaldo Maduro, "Artistic Creativity and Aging in India," *The International Journal of Aging and Human Development* 5, no. 4 (1974): 303-329.

[18] G. Cohen (2006): 8.

[19] Shinobu Kitayama, Martha K. Berg, and William J. Chopik, "Culture and Well-being in Late Adulthood: Theory and Evidence," *American Psychologist* 75, no. 4 (2020): 567-576.

[20] For example, see research by Lijuan Chen, Max Alston, and Wei Guo, "The Influence of Social Support on Loneliness and Depression Among Older Elderly People in China: Coping Styles as Mediators," *Journal of Community Psychology* 47, no. 5 (2019): 1235-1245. Jianghong Liu, Gary Lewis, and Lois Evans, "Understanding Aggressive Behaviour Across the Lifespan," *Journal of Psychiatric and Mental Health Nursing* 20, no. 2 (2013): 156-168. Glenn R. Marks and Susan K. Lutgendorf, "Perceived Health Competence and Personality Factors Differentially Predict Health Behaviors in Older Adults," *Journal of Aging and Health* 11, no. 2 (1999): 221-239. Marciana L. Popescu, Rene Drumm, Smita Dewan, and Corneliu Rusu, "Childhood Victimization and Its Impact on Coping Behaviors for Victims of Intimate Partner Violence," *Journal of Family Violence* 25, no. 6 (2010): 575-585. Natalie G. Regier and Patricia A. Parmelee, "The Stability of Coping Strategies in Older Adults with Osteoarthritis and the Ability of These Strategies to Predict Changes in Depression, Disability, and Pain," *Aging & Mental Health* 19, no. 12 (2015): 1113-1122. Carolyn Schwartz, Janice Bell Meisenhelder, Yunsheng Ma, and George Reed, "Altruistic Social Interest Behaviors are Associated with Better Mental Health," *Psychosomatic Medicine* 65, no. 5 (2003): 778-785.

[21] Benjamin Cornwell, Edward O. Laumann, and L. Philip Schumm, "The Social Connectedness of Older Adults: A National Profile," *American Sociological Review* 73, no. 2 (2008): 185-203. Miya Narushima, "A Gaggle of Raging Grannies: The Empowerment of Older Canadian Women Through Social Activism," *International Journal of Lifelong Education* 23, no. 1 (2004): 23-42.

[22] Michael W. Pratt, Gail Golding, and William J. Hunter, "Aging as Ripening: Character and Consistency of Moral Judgment in Young, Mature, and Older adults," *Human Development* 26, no. 5 (1983): 277-288.

[23] Simon McNair, Yasmina Okan, Constantinos Hadjichristidis, and Wändi Bruine de Bruin, "Age Differences in Moral Judgment: Older Adults are More Deontological than Younger Adults," *Journal of Behavioral Decision Making* 32, no. 1 (2019): 47-60.

[24] Julia Skelly, "Roy Henry Vickers," *The Canadian Encyclopedia*, 13 April 2018, *Historica Canada*. Accessed January 4, 2023, https://www.thecanadianencyclopedia.ca/en/article/roy-henry-vickers. Roy Henry Vickers, "Artist Biography," *Roy Henry Vickers Gallery* (2023). Accessed January 4, 2023, https://royhenryvickers.com/pages/artist-biography#:~:text=Roy%20studied%20traditional%20First%20Nations%20art%20and%20design,and%20contemporary%2C%20old%20and%20new%2C%20personal%20and%20universal. Roy Henry Vickers, "Life Lessons in Mindfulness," presentation at *The Heart-Mind Conference*, June, 2013, Vancouver, Canada. Accessed March 3, 2021, https://www.youtube.com/watch?v=UsiWudbaP-Q.

[25] Roy Henry Vickers, "Roy Henry Vickers Inspires National ASA in Victoria, Interview by Barbara Kermode-Scott," *Canadian Family Physician* 45 (1999): 2593-2601. World Council of Indigenous people, "Solemn Declaration," *UHM Library Digital Image Collections*. Accessed January 3, 2023, https://digital.library.manoa.hawaii.edu/items/show/31240.

[26] R. H. Vickers, *Canadian Family Physician* 45 (1999): 2595.

[27] The Editors of Encyclopedia Britannica, "Maggie Kuhn," *Encyclopedia Britannica*, 30 July 2022. Accessed January 4, 2023, https://www.britannica.com/biography/Maggie-Kuhn.

[28] Paul's Pantry – Neighbors Feeding Neighbors, "Our Founder." Accessed December 20, 2022. https://www.paulspantry.org/our-founder/

[29] For more information see, Bill McKibben, "Bill McKibben – Author.Educator.Environmentalist." Accessed January 5, 2023, http://billmckibben.com/index.html. Third Act, "Third Act." Accessed January 5, 2023, https://thirdact.org/. Judy Woodruff, "Bill McKibben, Environmentalist, Founder of Third Act - Brief but Spectacular," *PBS News Hour*. Accessed January 5, 2023, https://www.pbs.org/newshour/brief/430904/bill-mckibben

[30] NHK World - Japan, "The Toy Doctor – Zero Waste Life," July 2, 2021, educational video, 15:00, https://www3.nhk.or.jp/nhkworld/en/ondemand/video/2093003/ Osamu Sawaji, "The Joy of Fixing Toys," *Highlighting Japan*, August 2020: 20-21. Accessed August 1, 2023 at https://www.gov-online.go.jp/pdf/hlj/20200801/20-21.pdf

[31] For example, see works by Paul Connett, *The Zero Waste Solution: Untrashing the Planet One Community at a Time* (White River, Vermont: Chelsea Green Publishing, 2013). Atiq Zaman and Tahmina Ahsan, *Zero-Waste: Reconsidering Waste Management for the Future* (Philadelphia, PA: Routledge, 2019).

[32] NHK World – Japan (July 2, 2021).

[33] Darlene Donloe, *Gordon Parks* (Los Angeles, CA: Holloway House Publishing, 1993). Gordon Parks, *A Hungry Heart: A Memoir* (New York: Simon and Schuster, 2005). Gordon Parks, *Voices in the Mirror: An Autobiography* (New York: Broadway Books, 2005).

[34] Gwen Everett and Joann Moser, *African American Masters: Highlights from the Smithsonian American Art Museum* (Washington, D.C. and New York: Smithsonian American Art Museum in association with Harry N. Abrams, Inc., 2003).

[35] The Gordon Parks Museum, "Gordon Park's History and Time-Line" (The Gordon Parks Museum, Fort Scott Community College, Fort Scott, KS). Accessed January 6, 2023 https://www.gordonparkscenter.org/gordon-parks.

[36] Gordon Parks, *Flash Photography* (New York: Grosset,1947). Gordon Parks, *Camera Portraits: The Techniques and Principles of Documentary Portraiture* (Rockford, IL: Watts, 1948).

[37] Gordon Parks, *Eyes with Winged Thoughts: Poems and Photographs* (New York: Simon and Schuster, 2007). Gordon Parks and Philip Brookman, *Half Past Autumn: A Retrospective* (New York: Bulfinch Press, 1997). Craig Rice, *Half Past Autumn: The Life and Works of Gordon Parks* (New York: HBO Studios, 2000).

CHAPTER TWELVE – EPILOGUE: TELL ME THAT STORY AGAIN!

[1] Walt Whitman, "Youth, Day, Old Age and Night," *Leaves of Grass* (In the public domain, 1881-1882):180.

[2] A translation of the Latin phrase, "Ut est rerum omnium magister usus," attributed to the general and statesman Julius Caesar in his *Commentarii de Bello Civili (Commentaries on the Civil War),* about Roman military and political events of occurring in 49—48 BC, and published in 46 BC.

[3] For example, see works by the following: Peta S. Cook, "Continuity, Change and Possibility in Older Age: Identity and Ageing-as-Discovery," *Journal of Sociology* 54, no. 2 (2018): 178-190. Susan Feldman, and Linsey Howie, "Looking Back, Looking Forward: Reflections on Using a Life History Review Tool with Older People," *Journal of Applied Gerontology* 28, no. 5 (2009): 621-637. Susan Hupkens, Anja Machielse, Marleen Goumans, and Peter Derkx, "Meaning in Life of Older Persons: An Integrative Literature Review," *Nursing Ethics* 25, no. 8 (2018): 973-991.

[4] See reports by, Michael Nahm, Bruce Greyson, Emily Williams Kelly, and Erlendur Haraldsson, "Terminal Lucidity: A Review and a Case Collection," *Archives of Gerontology and Geriatrics* 55, no. 1 (2012): 138-142. Shared Crossing Research Initiative, "The Spectrum of End-of-Life Experiences: A Tool for Advancing Death Education," *OMEGA-Journal of Death and Dying* (2022): 00302228211052342. Jeanne A. Teresi, Mildred Ramirez, Julie Ellis, Amil Tan, Elizabeth Capezuti, Stephanie Silver, Gabriel Boratgis et al., "Reports About Paradoxical Lucidity from Health Care Professionals: A Pilot Study," *Journal of Gerontological Nursing* 49, no. 1 (2023): 18-26.

[5] For example, see the following works: Jerome Bruner, *Acts of Meaning* (Cambridge, MA: Harvard University Press,1990). Jerome Bruner, "The Narrative Construction of Reality," *Critical Inquiry* 18, no. 1 (1991): 1-21. Jerome S. Bruner, "On Perceptual Readiness," *Psychological Review* 64, no. 2 (1957): 123. Batja Mesquita, Lisa Feldman Barrett, and Eliot R. Smith, eds., *The Mind in Context* (New York, NY: Guilford Press, 2010).

[6] For example, see the following works: Stephen C. Ainlay and Donald L. Redfoot, "Aging and Identity-in-the-World: A Phenomenological Analysis," *The International Journal of Aging and Human Development* 15, no. 1 (1983): 1-16. Michael Bavidge, "Feeling One's Age: A Phenomenology of Aging," Geoffrey Scarre (ed.) *The Palgrave Handbook of the Philosophy of Aging* (London: Palgrave Macmillan, 2016): 207-224. Nelson Goodman, "The Way the World Is," *The Review of Metaphysics* (1960): 48-56.

[7] Roy Henry Vickers, "Artist Biography," *Roy Henry Vickers Gallery* (2023). Accessed January 4, 2023, https://royhenryvickers.com/pages/artist-biography#:~:text=Roy%20studied%20traditional%20First%20Nations%20art%20and%20design,and%20contemporary%2C%20old%20and%20new%2C%20personal%20and%20universal. Roy Henry Vickers, "Life Lessons in Mindfulness," presentation at *The Heart-Mind Conference*, June, 2013, Vancouver, Canada. Accessed March 3, 2021, https://www.youtube.com/watch?v=UsiWudbaP-Q.

[8] Victoria Jicha, "Personal Communication to Dean D. VonDras" (October, 2020).

[9] Helane S. Rosenberg and William Trusheim, "Creative Transformations: How Visual artists, Musicians, and Dancers Use Mental Imagery in Their Work," *Imagery: Current Perspectives* (1989): 55-75.

[10] Gary T. Reker and Paul T. R. Wong, "Personal Meaning in Life and Psychosocial Adaptation in the Later Years," in P. T. P. Wong, ed., *The Human Quest for Meaning: Theories, Research, and Applications* (New York: Routledge): 433-456.

[11] Ann S. Masten, Karin M. Best, and Norman Garmezy, "Resilience and Development: Contributions from the Study of Children who Overcome Adversity," *Development and Psychopathology* 2, no. 4 (1990): 425-444. Steven M. Southwick and Dennis S. Charney, *Resilience: The Science of Mastering Life's Greatest Challenges* (Cambridge: Cambridge University Press, 2018).

[12] Scott F. Madey and Dean D. VonDras, *Music, Wellness, and Aging: Defining, Directing, and Celebrating Life* (Cambridge: Cambridge University Press, 2021).

[13] Lewis Piaget Shanks, "Theophile Gautier," *The Sewanee Review* 20, no. 2 (1912): 167-174.

[14] Lee Newitt, "The Journey's Hero," in P. Worth, ed., *Positive Psychology Across the Lifespan: An Existential Perspective* (New York, NY: Routledge, 2022): 61-78.

[15] NME Editors, "The Beatles and The Doors' Music Played on Mars During NASA Mission," *NME*, 1August 17, 2012. Accessed, May 22, 2023 at https://www.nme.com/news/music/the-beatles-177-1254283.

[16] Houston Methodist Editors, "Center for Performing Arts Medicine," *Houston Methodist*. Accessed, 20 July 2023 at https://www.houstonmethodist.org/performing-arts/

[17] Jeff Balke, "Musical Medicine: Hospital Concert Series Just What the Doctor Ordered," *Houston Press*, October 11, 2017. Accessed, June 5, 2023, at https://www.houstonpress.com/music/find-your-next-concert-in-the-lobby-at-methodist-hospital-9865482.

[18] Britni R. McAshan, "Houston Methodist Employees' Art Helps Patients Navigate the Emergency Department," *TMC* (Texas Medical Center), November 1, 2018. Accessed, July 20, 2023 at https://www.tmc.edu/news/2018/11/houston-methodist-employees-art-helps-patients-navigate-the-emergency-department/the pARTnership movement. Web-Editors, "Success Stories: Houston Methodist (Houston, TX)," *the pARTnership movement*, n.d. Accessed, July 20, 2023 at https://www.partnershipmovement.org/partnership-inspiration/success-stories/houston-methodist-houston-tx

[19] Shay Thornton Kulha, J. Todd Frazier, Jennifer Townsend, Elizabeth Laguaite, and Virginia Gray, "'An Anchor in a Stormy Sea': An Arts in Health Project for Healthcare Staff During COVID-19," *Journal of Applied Arts & Health* 12, no. 3 (2023): 353-366.

[20] Robin Soslow, "Discover Seismique, Houston's Exciting Immersive Art Experience for All Ages," *Chron*, May 14, 2023. Accessed, July 21, 2023 at https://www.chron.com/culture/arts/article/seismique-17905912.php

[21] Jennifer Ebert, "Small Backyard Landscaping Ideas – 15 Clever Designs for Tiny Spaces," *Homes & Gardens*, May 9, 2022. Accessed, July 21, 2023 at https://www.homesandgardens.com/ideas/small-yard-landscaping-ideas. Sarah Price, "How to Create an Immersive Garden," *Gardens Illustrated*, November 23, 2015. Accessed, July 20, 2023 at https://www.gardensillustrated.com/garden-design/how-to-create- Cooper an-immersive-garden

[22] Clare Marcus and Marni Barnes, eds. *Healing Gardens: Therapeutic Benefits and Design Recommendations*, Vol. 4. (Hoboken, NJ: John Wiley & Sons, 1999).

[23] ACGA Executive Board, "The Healing Power of Simple Gardening," *Community Gardening, The American Community Gardening Association*, Vol. 26, no. 1 (2023): 4.

[24] New Horizons International Music Association, "Concept and Philosophy," n.d. Accessed July 21, 2023 at https://newhorizonsmusic.org/Concept_and_Philosophy

[25] Roy Ernst, "Music and Your Health," Workshop Presentation in Dayton Ohio (April, 2011). Accessed July 21, 2023 at https://newhorizonsmusic.starchapter.com/images/downloads/Documents/music_and_health.pdf

[26] Drum Corps Associates, "The Finest Drum & Bugle Corps in the US and Canada," n.d. Accessed August 4, 2023 at https://dcacorps.org/about-drum-corps-associates. National Band Association, "Community Bands," n.d., Accessed August 4, 2023 at https://nationalbandassociation.org/about/community-bands/

[27] For example, see reports by the following: Tuulikki Laes, "Empowering Later Adulthood Music Education: A Case Study of a Rock Band for Third-Age Learners," *International Journal of Music Education* 33, no. 1 (2015): 51-65. Helen O'Shea, "'Get Back to Where You Once Belonged!'1 The Positive Creative Impact of a Refresher Course for 'Baby-Boomer' Rock Musicians," *Popular Music* 31, no. 2 (2012): 199-215.

[28] Barbershop Harmony Society, "A Truly American Artform, Barbershop Harmony is Music," n.d. Accessed August 4, 2023 at https://www.barbershop.org/about. Chorus America, "About Chorus America," n.d. Accessed August 3, 2023 at https://chorusamerica.org/about. International Federation for Choral Music, "IFCM: "Volunteers Connecting Our Choral World," n.d. Accessed August 4, 2023 at https://ifcm.net/about-us/mission

[29] See for example, reports by, Quin Campbell, Sally Bodkin-Allen, and Nicola Swain, "Group Singing Improves both Physical and Psychological Wellbeing in People With and Without Chronic Health Conditions: A Narrative Review," *Journal of Health Psychology* 27, no. 8 (2022): 1897-1912. Julene K. Johnson, Anita L. Stewart, Michael Acree, Anna M. Nápoles, Jason D. Flatt, Wendy B. Max, and Steven E. Gregorich, "A Community Choir Intervention to Promote Well-being Among Diverse Older Adults: Results from the Community of Voices Trial," *The Journals of Gerontology: Series B* 75, no. 3 (2020): 549-559. Julene K. Johnson, Jukka Louhivuori, Anita L. Stewart, Asko Tolvanen, Leslie Ross, and Pertti Era, "Quality of Life (QOL) of Older Adult Community Choral Singers in Finland," *International Psychogeriatrics* 25, no. 7 (2013): 1055-1064. C. Reagon, N. Gale, R. Dow, I. Lewis, and R. Van Deursen, "Choir Singing and Health Status in People Affected by Cancer," *European Journal of Cancer Care* 26, no. 5 (2017): e12568. Elyse Williams, Genevieve A. Dingle, and Stephen Clift, "A Systematic Review of Mental Health and Wellbeing Outcomes of Group Singing for Adults with a Mental Health Condition," *European Journal of Public Health* 28, no. 6 (2018): 1035-1042. Also, see for example, reports by, J. Yoon Irons, David Sheffield, Freddie Ballington, and Donald E. Stewart, "A Systematic Review on the Effects of Group Singing on Persistent Pain in People with Long-term Health Conditions," *European Journal of Pain* 24, no. 1 (2020): 71-90. Ann Skingley, Sonia Page, Stephen Clift, Ian Morrison, Simon Coulton, Pauline Treadwell, Trish Vella-Burrows, Isobel Salisbury, and Matthew Shipton., ""Singing for Breathing": Participants' Perceptions of a Group Singing Programme for People with COPD," *Arts & Health* 6, no. 1 (2014): 59-74.

[30] V. Jicha, *The Flutist Quarterly, Vol. 46, No. 4: 20-24.*

31 Gary Glazner, "Sparking Creativity With Poetry: Alzheimer's Poetry Project," n.d. Accessed June 5, 2023 at https://www.alzpoetry.com. Gary M. Glazner, *Dementia Arts: Celebrating Creativity in Elder Care* (Baltimore, MD: Health Professions Press, 2014).

32 Felix Geser, Kurt A. Jellinger, Lisa Fellner, Gregor K. Wenning, Deniz Yilmazer-Hanke, and Johannes Haybaeck, "Emergent Creativity in Frontotemporal Dementia," *Journal of Neural Transmission* 128 (2021): 279-293. Bruce L. Miller and Craig E. Hou, "Portraits of Artists: Emergence of Visual Creativity in Dementia," *Archives of Neurology* 61, no. 6 (2004): 842-844.

33 For example, see works by, Jackie Ashley, Debbie Michaels, Simon Bell, Iris Von Sass Hyde, Carole Connelly, Anna Knight, Quentin Bruckland et al., *Art Therapy with Neurological Conditions* (London: Jessica Kingsley Publishers, 2015). Crystal Ehresman, "From Rendering to Remembering: Art Therapy for People with Alzheimer's Disease," *International Journal of Art Therapy* 19, no. 1 (2014): 43-51. Christine Jonas-Simpson, Gail Mitchell, Sherry Dupuis, Lesley Donovan, and Pia Kontos, "Free to Be: Experiences of Arts-Based Relational Caring in a Community Living and Thriving with Dementia," *Dementia* 21, no. 1 (2022): 61-76. Irfan Manji, Tanita Cepalo, Sergio Ledesma, and Pascal Fallavollita, "Personhood, QOL, and Well-being in People with Dementia undergoing Creative Arts-based Therapies: A Scoping Review," *Creativity Research Journal* (2023): 1-23. Roslyn G. Poulos, Sally Marwood, Damian Harkin, Simon Opher, Stephen Clift, Andrew MD Cole, Joel Rhee, Kirsty Beilharz, and Christopher J. Poulos, "Arts on Prescription for Community-Dwelling Older People With a Range of Health and Wellness Needs," *Health & Social Care in the Community* 27, no. 2 (2019): 483-492. Paula Rylatt, "The Benefits of Creative Therapy for People with Dementia," *Nursing Standard* 26, no. 33 (2012).

34 For example, François Boller, Elena Sinforiani, and Anna Mazzucchi, "Preserved Painting Abilities After a Stroke. The Case of Paul-Elie Gernez," *Functional Neurology* 20, no. 4 (2005): 151-156. B. L. Miller and C. E. Hou, *Archives of Neurology* 61, no. 6 (2004): 842-844. G. D. Schott, "Pictures as a Neurological Tool: Lessons from Enhanced and Emergent Artistry in Brain Disease," *Brain* 135, no. 6 (2012): 1947-1963.

35 For example, National Arts Council of Singapore, "The Arts Plan," n.d. Accessed, 5 June 2023 at https://www.nac.gov.sg/resources/toolkits-and-guides/community-engagement/guide-to-impacting-communities-through-the-arts-(2021).

36 For example, see the following websites: Manhattan Arts International, "The Healing Power of Ars and Artists," n.d. Accessed, 5 June 2023 at https://www.healing-power-of-art.org/art-and-healing-organizations/. Mind in Kingston, "Community Arts Therapy," n.d. Accessed, 5 June, 2023 at https://nationalguild.org/ Community Art therapy – Mind in Kingston. National Guild for Community Arts Education, "About the Guild," n.d. Accessed, 5 June, 2023 at https://nationalguild.org/about/about-the-guildhttps://nationalguild.org/about/about-the-guild

[37] There are many ways to be creative and to leave a legacy of one's artful and imaginative expressions, and includes everything from writing one's autobiography to learning to play the xylophone, as well as activities such as developing a catalogue of plants discovered on hikes in the woods, keeping a diary or personal journal, developing a portfolio of paintings, photographs, or drawings, creating a library of design plans for garden sculptures, making community maps that distinguish landmarks of personal interest or trips one has taken, maintaining a scrapbook of family accomplishments and activities, keeping a collection of special things or objects, creating an encyclopedia of clichés or special phrases, writing your own family recipe book, writing original songs or music, writing a memoir or family history, or leaving a catalogue of special activities that one may have enjoyed—there is no limit to what you might undertake to express your creativity and to leave a legacy that celebrates your living and offers a message of hope for others.

[38] Emma Taggart, "How to Make a Zine: A Guide to Self-Publishing Your Own Miniature Magazine," *My Modern Met,* September 7, 2021. Accessed August 21, 2023 at https://mymodernmet.com/how-to-make-a-zine/

[39] L. Tornstam, *Journal of Transpersonal Psychology* 43, no. 2 (2011): 166-180

[40] Walt Whitman, "Twilight," *Leaves of Grass* (in the public domain, 1891-1892): 454.

Index

www.ingramcontent.com/pod-product-compliance
Lightning Source LLC
Chambersburg PA
CBHW061717270326
41928CB00011B/2017